The DASH Diet for Every Day

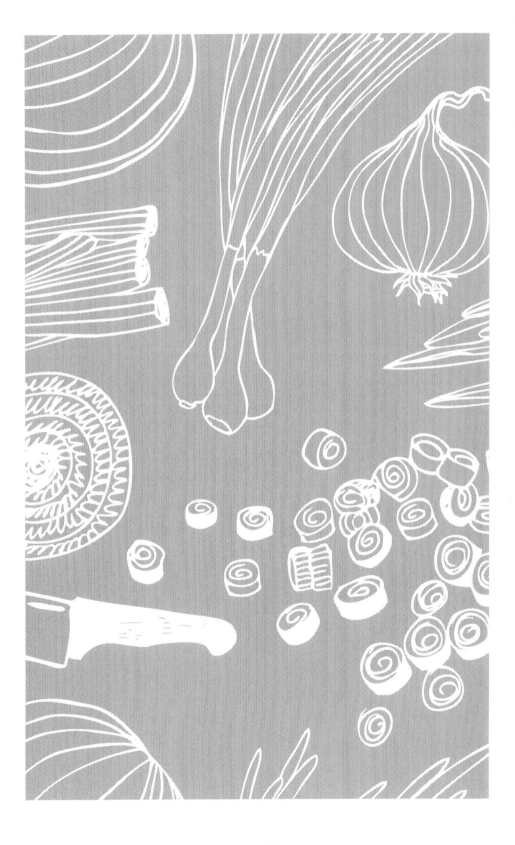

The DASH Diet for Every Day

4 WEEKS OF DASH DIET RECIPES & MEAL PLANS TO LOSE WEIGHT & IMPROVE HEALTH

TELAMON
PRESS

Contents

Introduction

So, you want to lose those extra inches and get healthy. You've done your research and come across dozens of diet plans that promise results. You're asking yourself, "Which one is the right one?" Maybe you've tried a few diets and found that some of them can, in fact, help you lose weight—if you manage to stick with them. There's the rub: A lot of diets out there are just too hard to follow. They ask you to deprive and starve yourself, eat weird foods, follow convoluted instructions, take expensive pills and potions, or exercise like a gym rat. A lot of them aren't backed up by solid science. And a lot of them aren't actually all that good for your health.

But there is a proven, acclaimed, sustainable way to lose fat and gain wellness: the DASH diet. Not just a diet, it's a rewarding, lifelong style of eating that's endorsed by the National Institutes of Health and the United States Department of Agriculture. The DASH diet is a commonsense plan that shifts you away from saturated fat, cholesterol, and refined sugar and toward lean meats, fish, poultry, low-fat dairy, fruits, vegetables, and whole grains. Most importantly, though, it slashes your sodium intake. If you've got hypertension (high blood pressure), diabetes, osteoporosis, or kidney disease; if you're at risk for heart disease; if you want to get rid of your spare tire or thunder thighs; or if you're just looking for a way to eat better and feel better, the DASH diet is for you.

In Part One of this book, you'll learn in a nutshell what makes the DASH diet so effective at reducing blood pressure and burning fat and why it's so easy to follow. Then, in Part Two, you'll cut straight to the chase: how to work the program. The key to DASH dieting is planning—specifically, meal planning. Planning your meals and your daily and weekly menus is essential because it all but eliminates your risk of falling off the wagon. If you know ahead of time what you're going to eat, you don't have to make any decisions when you're hungry. That means you'll make fewer bad decisions. And when you go into your days and weeks with a preset eating plan, you always have lots of delicious food on hand. That means you're less likely to be tempted by quick hunger fixes like microwave meals, junk snacks, and fast food. You'll still face a lot of challenges, but every chapter of this book is packed with tips and suggestions on adjusting to, staying with, and enjoying the DASH way of eating.

Part Two makes it simple for you to succeed with the DASH diet by laying out a practical, no-hassle four-week meal plan that, after a few days of adjustment, will painlessly fit into your hectic routine. That's right: This book not only explains the DASH diet and tells you what to do, it actually teaches you how to follow the diet. It shows you exactly how to put the meal-planning guidelines into action.

Once you've got the meal-planning tools, Part Three gives you the delicious nuts and bolts of the DASH diet: more than sixty recipes. Even if you're not much of a cook, even if you've never turned on your stove, these quick, fuss-free recipes aren't intimidating. And if you do know your way around the kitchen—blindfolded—these fresh, vibrant dishes will open your eyes to the potential of healthful cuisine. Whether you're a rookie or an ace, you'll be happy to find that the DASH recipes use affordable, familiar ingredients that you can buy in your regular supermarket. The uncomplicated, timesaving techniques make everyday meal prep smooth and speedy. Plus, cooking tips galore will save you money, time, and stress.

With smart meal planning, DASH is a diet that you can really work with, and that will really work for you.

Getting Started

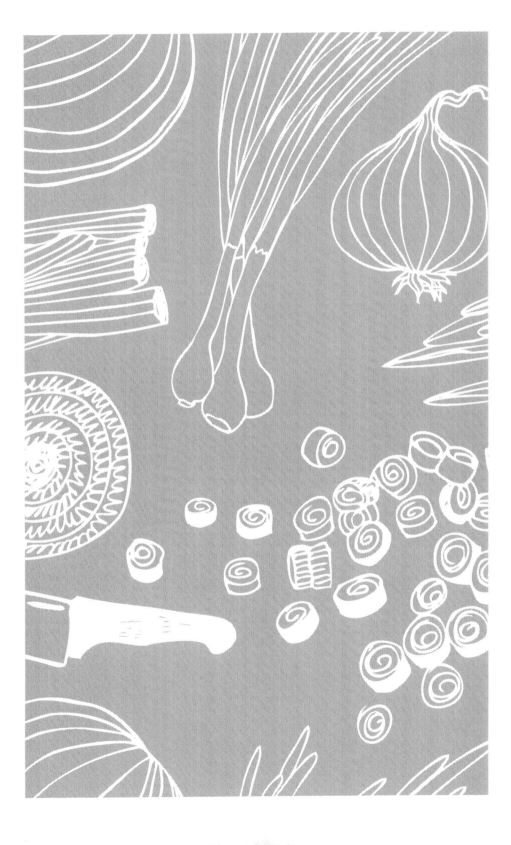

CHAPTER ONE

DASH Diet Basics

The DASH diet is a great tool for losing weight, but it wasn't invented as a weight-loss program. *DASH* stands for Dietary Approaches to Stop Hypertension, and the plan is as scientifically substantial as its name. It was developed by a group of researchers that included experts from elite institutions such as Harvard Medical School, Johns Hopkins Medical Center, and Duke University School of Medicine, and the work was funded by the federal government's National Institutes of Health (NIH). The goal was to design a diet that would help people suffering from hypertension to lower their blood pressure, and DASH does so, brilliantly.

But there's more to it. Since 1993, when DASH was created, scientists have found that the diet not only reduces blood pressure in a matter of weeks, but it also brings down cholesterol levels. Plus, people who follow the plan are at lower risk of heart disease and heart failure, stroke, certain cancers, diabetes, osteoporosis, and kidney problems. On top of all those health benefits, DASH is recognized as an excellent weight-loss program. So even if you don't have high blood pressure or low bone density or another health problem, DASH is an outstanding choice for slimming down.

There's no doubt that DASH is as safe, effective, and healthful a weight-loss and blood pressure–reduction program as you can find. In each of the three years *U.S. News & World Report* has ranked diet plans, DASH earned the top spot as the best overall diet. DASH also has many prestigious endorsements from organizations that include the National Heart, Lung, and Blood Institute (part of the NIH), the United States Department of Agriculture (USDA), the American Heart Association (AHA), and the Mayo Clinic. What more could you ask for?

WHAT IS THE DASH DIET?

Simply put, the DASH diet is common sense. Eating right is all there is to it. That's it. There are no rigid rules to obey, no complicated steps to follow, no hoops to jump through, no bells and whistles to confuse you. Just eat the foods that are good for you. Without realizing it, your mom probably told you to eat the DASH way. The only difference is that now there's science to back up what she knew all along.

All you do on DASH is pay attention to what you're eating, and eat good food in intelligent portions. That means eating lots of fresh vegetables, fruit, whole grains, and legumes (beans), and reasonable amounts of lean meat, poultry, seafood, low-fat dairy, and good fats like nuts. It also means cutting out processed foods such as frozen dinners, sugary sodas and sweets, salty snacks, refined grains, and fatty meats.

What you end up with are balanced, reasonable-size meals that deliver a lot of flavor and variety. This diet pumps you full of nutrients, keeps you feeling full all day, and helps you lose weight. You have plenty of energy for moderate exercise (thirty minutes, three times a week, if you can) that will make you feel even better. The exercise, plus the plentiful potassium, calcium, magnesium, fiber, and protein, and the low levels of sodium in your food help bring down your blood pressure. When you start seeing the results of DASH, whether on your waistline or in your doctor's office, you'll be hooked.

WHY FOLLOW THE DASH DIET?

Reason One: You don't feel deprived.

Five or six times a day, you eat foods that keep you feeling full until it's time to eat again. In fact, you might find it a little difficult to eat as much and as often as DASH recommends, even if you're eating fewer calories than you're used to. The secret lies in what you're eating. Fruit, vegetables, and whole grains packed with fiber fill you up and slow down your digestion, while high-protein foods such as lean meat, poultry, fish, and low-fat dairy products stimulate the release of a hormone that makes you feel satisfied and suppresses your desire to eat more. And you don't even have to give up all the "bad" foods that you love. Go ahead and indulge your guilty cravings every so often. Eat out at restaurants and nibble at parties.

Reason Two: You don't feel tired.

Recommended DASH foods boost your energy level and keep it up for hours. You won't be pigging out on the junk food that causes your blood sugar levels to spike and then plunge, leaving you fatigued. Feeling great, not to mention looking great and seeing great health and fitness results pretty quickly, will keep you motivated.

Reason Three: It's easy.

The changes you're making in your diet don't have to be extreme and awkward. DASH gives you so many food options that you may keep eating a lot of the dishes you've always loved. You may even re-create your favorite restaurant and store-bought standbys in healthier forms. Your family, even your kids, may eat the same things you're eating, so you don't have to shop for and prepare separate meals. And if you have specific dietary needs—gluten-free, vegetarian, vegan, kosher, halal, or something else—you can easily adapt the DASH diet to fit your lifestyle.

Reason Four: It's free.

There are no official DASH-branded foods, gadgets, or publications to buy. You don't have to pay a monthly fee to join a group and gain access to DASH secrets. The choice is yours whether to invest in a gym membership, fitness classes, or exercise gear. Of course, you do have to buy your groceries, but that's nothing new; you'll just be buying different groceries. And DASH is so flexible that you may easily spend less at the supermarket than you were spending before.

Reason Five: There's no risk.

You're not risking any money (see Reason Four), and you're not risking your health. DASH follows the nutritional recommendations of virtually every respected health organization, from the United States government to the American Diabetes Association, and adheres to the nutritional principles embraced by the medical community in general. You get plenty of everything you need, nothing you shouldn't have, and just enough of everything in between.

DASH researchers have found that the program is a more powerful tool for reducing blood pressure and improving heart health than taking a pill. Heart-healthful supplements such as calcium, potassium, and magnesium have virtually no impact if you take them without cutting back on processed foods. In addition, some studies have shown that the DASH diet can bring down blood pressure as effectively as antihypertensive medication. Some doctors actually prescribe the DASH diet instead of blood pressure medication for people who aren't at high risk of stroke or heart attack.

THE DASH DIET AND WEIGHT LOSS

The key to losing weight is *calorie deficit*: Take in fewer calories than you burn, and you lose weight. For example, if you want to lose one pound of fat in a week, you've got to burn 3,500 more calories than you eat—a deficit of 500 calories a day—or eat fewer calories, or both. In one form or another, every diet plan uses this technique. But if you want to get healthier as well as thinner, and if you want to keep those pounds off once you've shed them, DASH is the ideal program. The secret to healthful, lasting weight loss is choosing the right foods, and DASH makes that easy to do.

Before you start any weight-loss program, consult your health care provider about your health limitations and ask him or her to help you set a healthful weight goal. Your health provider can also help you figure out how many calories you should eat each day and what kinds of exercise you should do to put your weight-loss plan into action. Reliable online sources, such as the Centers for Disease Control and Prevention's "Healthy Weight" web page (http://www.cdc.gov/healthyweight/index.html) and WebMD's "Weight Loss and Diet Plans" web page (http://www.webmd.com/diet/calc-bmi-plus), can also help you determine your healthful weight, calculate how many calories you've been eating on average, and set the caloric and nutritional parameters of a sound, personalized weight-loss and blood pressure–reduction plan. DASH will do the rest by empowering you to choose foods that will help you reach—and remain at—your target weight while satisfying both your nutritional needs and your taste buds.

The DASH program laid out in this book is a 2,000-calories-per-day diet. If your calorie requirement for weight loss or weight management is lower or higher, adjust your eating plan up or down: To get fewer calories, eat one or two fewer servings of both grains and fruits each day. You may also replace some of the higher-calorie DASH foods with lower-calorie choices in the same nutritional category—say, snapper instead of salmon. Conversely, if you need to take in more than 2,000 calories a day, eat more fruits and vegetables; if that's not enough, add more grains. Or choose that salmon instead of the snapper.

DASH makes sense for weight loss because it boosts your chances of success by letting you eat a wide variety of foods that will satisfy your appetite, curb your cravings, and keep you feeling full all day. It calls for moderate rather than radical changes to your diet and keeps your metabolism burning steadily. You'll be healthier than ever and will feel better as well as look better every day. And by turning you on to a more healthful long-term way of eating, DASH will help you maintain your new figure after you reach your target weight.

DASH DIET GUIDELINES

The DASH diet can be distilled into several straightforward, common-sense guidelines:

- Increase your intake of whole grains.
- Increase your intake of vegetables and fruits.
- Increase your intake of lean protein.
- Increase your intake of low-fat dairy foods.
- Decrease your intake of cholesterol and saturated fat, and eliminate trans fat.
- Decrease your intake of red meat and processed meat products.
- Decrease your intake of sugar, high-fructose corn syrup, and sugar substitutes.
- Decrease your intake of alcohol and caffeine.
- Decrease your daily sodium intake to the range of 1,500 mg–2,300 mg.

Following these guidelines, along with limiting your calories, ensures not only that you're on your way to your ideal body size and blood pressure, but also that you're on your way to feeding your body the best possible combination of nutrients for overall good health. The following table outlines what you should shoot for.

DASH Diet Daily Nutrition Recommendations	
Calcium	1,250 mg
Carbohydrates	55 percent of calories
Cholesterol	less than 150 mg
Fiber	30 grams
Magnesium	500 mg
Potassium	less than 4,700 mg
Protein	18 percent of calories
Saturated fat	6 percent of calories
Sodium	less than 2,300 mg (1,500 mg recommended)
Total fat	27 percent of calories
Vitamin B_{12}	at least 2.4 mg

On a 2,000-calorie-per-day diet, you can make sure you get all these nutrients—and all of the delicious food you want—by distributing those calories across eight groups of foods. Here's what you should eat.

DASH Diet Food Guidelines (Based on 2,000 Calories per Day)			
Food Group	Serving	Examples of One Serving	Approximate Daily Total
Whole grains	7–8 per day	½ cup (cooked) brown rice, whole-grain pasta, or whole-grain hot cereal; 1 slice multigrain bread; 1 ounce high-fiber cold cereal	6½ ounces

DASH Diet Food Guidelines (Based on 2,000 Calories per Day)			
Vegetables	4–5 per day	½ cup (cut-up) raw or cooked vegetables; 1 cup (raw) leafy vegetables	2½ cups
Fruits	4–5 per day	½ cup (cut-up) fresh or frozen fruit; 1 medium piece handheld fruit; ¼ cup dried fruit	2½ cups
Nonfat and low-fat dairy products	2–3 per day	1 cup milk or yogurt; 1½ ounces cheese	3 cups
Lean meats, poultry, seafood, and eggs	No more than 2 per day	3 ounces lean meat, poultry, or seafood; 1 egg; 6 egg whites	5½ ounces lean meat, poultry, or seafood
Fats and oils (at least 80 percent mono- and polyunsaturated fat; no more than 20 percent saturated fat)	No more than 2 per day	1 teaspoon tub margarine; 1 teaspoon vegetable oil; 1 tablespoon light mayonnaise; 2 tablespoons light salad dressing	Varies, depending on high-, medium-, or low-fat source
Nuts, seeds, and legumes	4–5 per week	⅓ cup or 1½ ounces nuts; 2 tablespoons unsalted natural nut butter; 2 tablespoons or ½ ounce seeds; ½ cup (cooked) beans or peas	Varies, depending on the food

DASH Diet Food Guidelines (Based on 2,000 Calories per Day)			
Sweets and added sugars (including alcoholic beverages)	No more than 5 per week; no more than 2 drinks per day for men or 1 drink per day for women	1 tablespoon sugar; 1 tablespoon jelly or jam; ½ cup sorbet or gelatin; 1 cup home-made lemonade	Varies, depending on the food

If 2,000 calories a day is too much or too little for your personal weight-loss needs, you may adjust the plan. Here are a couple of examples of how to do it.

DASH Diet Eating Guidelines for 1,600 and 2,600 Calories per Day		
Food Group	Servings for 1,600 Calories per Day	Servings for 2,600 Calories per Day
Whole grains	6 per day	10–11 per day
Vegetables	3–4 per day	5–6 per day
Fruits	4 per day	5–6 per day
Nonfat and low-fat dairy products	2–3 per day	3 per day
Fats and oils (at least 80 percent mono- and polyunsaturated fat; no more than 20 percent saturated fat)	2 per day	3 per day
Lean meats, poultry, seafood, and eggs	1–2 per day	2 per day
Nuts, seeds, and legumes	3 per week	1 per week
Sweets and added sugars (including alcoholic beverages)	0 per week	no more than 2 per week

DASH DIET FOOD GROUPS

One of the goals scientists aimed for when developing the DASH diet was to keep the focus on saying yes to eating all the right foods, instead of saying no to eating any of the wrong foods. DASH is designed for abundance, not deprivation. Nothing—*nothing*—is entirely off-limits. The DASH diet divides foods into eight groups, each of which contains "good" and "bad" choices. Choosing to eat the DASH-recommended foods from each group has distinct benefits for your weight-loss endeavors as well as for your blood pressure–reduction efforts and your overall health.

The original DASH diet was based on the USDA's 1992 food pyramid, which divided foods into six distinct groups to illustrate the government agency's recommendations for healthful eating. Ongoing research led the USDA to update its diet specifications in 2005, prompting the NIH to tweak the DASH guidelines. DASH still keeps pace with changing USDA findings, which were last updated in 2011. That year, the food pyramid was replaced by MyPlate, which simplifies the USDA's food groups into just five categories to present the latest recommendations.

Whole Grains

When selecting grains, think whole-grain pasta, bread, and similar products, and unrefined grains such as brown or wild rice, oats, barley, bulgur, and quinoa. Many of these grains may be used in place of white rice or cooked as a hot cereal for breakfast. They contain complex carbohydrates and fiber to keep you feeling full and energetic and plenty of vitamins and minerals that you need to be healthy.

Vegetables

Perhaps the most healthful foods you can eat, whether or not you're on the DASH diet, are dark leafy greens. But you should eat a wide variety of fiber- and nutrient-rich fresh vegetables in all different colors—everything from carrots, bell peppers, summer squash, tomatoes, and cauliflower to more green stuff such as broccoli, green beans, lettuces, asparagus, and celery. Your options are almost limitless. Be careful, though, with starchy vegetables such as potatoes, winter squash, and corn, which all quickly convert to sugar after you eat them. For information on legumes, such as dried beans, peas, and lentils, keep reading this list.

Fruits

Packed with vitamins, fruits contain a perfect combination of natural sugars and fiber, which prevents the sugars from entering your bloodstream too quickly. You name it, you may eat it, as long as it's fresh (or frozen without added sugar, high-fructose corn syrup, or other ingredients). One of the very few exceptions, if you're looking to lose weight, is high-fat, high-calorie avocado: Just one ounce counts as an entire fruit serving.

Lean Meats, Poultry, Seafood, and Eggs

Protein is essential for many bodily functions, and it helps curb hunger. You don't have to do away with red meat, just steer clear of the fatty cuts and go for the lean cuts. When buying poultry, opt for the breast and leave off the skin. Fish and eggs, especially egg whites, are your friends. Another great option is soy protein in the form of plain (not seasoned or flavored) tofu, tempeh, soy milk, and more. Be careful at the deli counter, though—many cold cuts contain additives such as salt, MSG, and even sugar.

Nonfat and Low-Fat Dairy Products

In their reduced-fat forms, milk, yogurt (especially Greek yogurt), low-sodium cottage cheese, and other low-sodium soft cheeses are wonderful additions to the DASH diet. They're rich in protein and calcium, as well as many vitamins, and they're a great cure for hunger pangs. Just be sure to go with the simplest forms, with no added fruit preserves or other sugars, salt, or commercial additives.

Nuts, Seeds, and Legumes

Vegetarians have long relied on nuts, seeds, and legumes as sources of protein and fiber. Legumes such as pinto and black beans, peas, and lentils are full of complex carbohydrates and minerals, while nuts and seeds contain the kinds of fat that are good for your heart. All three foods stick to your ribs, making them great additions when you're cutting back on calories. Note, however, that legumes don't fulfill all of your protein needs on their own. You need to eat them in combination with grains to get the protein profile your body needs.

Healthful Fats and Oils

To remain healthy, you must eat fat—the right kinds of fat, that is. Fat plays a crucial role in many bodily functions, and "good" fat actually helps control your cholesterol level. Grape-seed, avocado, and walnut oils are the best for you, but they may not be suitable to every recipe. No worries—extra-virgin olive oil, canola oil, and safflower oil are highly beneficial, too. Omega-3 fatty acids from fish are great for your heart. Make sure to choose healthful mono- and polyunsaturated fats, and use them in moderation to keep your calorie count down.

Sweets and Added Sugars

DASH allows you to eat sweets, in moderation. Sweets aren't considered a source of nutrition, but they're essential because having the occasional sugary treat helps keep you from feeling deprived and giving up on your diet. If you manage to save them for special occasions, they seem even more like a reward. When you do eat sweets, choose low-fat or nonfat options such as pure maple syrup, fruit-flavored gelatin, or sorbet. Because sugar is packed with empty calories, be careful to stick with the recommended portion sizes. Natural sugar substitutes such as stevia and xylitol are allowed to reduce calorie count and sugar intake, but they have their own downsides and should be limited. They don't give you license to increase the number of sweets servings you consume!

FOODS TO AVOID

Although DASH doesn't entirely forbid any particular food, it's a good idea to avoid certain foods that seriously deviate from the guidelines. If your goal is to cut back on calories, saturated and trans fat, sugar, sodium, and red meat, it's best to limit or entirely stay away from the especially bad stuff. Don't buy it, and if you've got any of it in your house, office, or car, get rid of it. This is only a partial list.

Beverages

- Coffee drinks with cream, whipped cream, sugar, or sweet flavorings
- Energy drinks
- Sugary or artificially sweetened sodas
- Sugary or artificially sweetened soft drinks, such as iced tea, lemonade, fruit "drinks" or "cocktails," and flavored waters

Processed Foods

- Artificial "cheese foods," such as American cheese, spray cheese, and cheese spreads
- Canned soups, stews, pastas, sauces, and gravies
- Frozen, boxed, or canned meals, entrées, soups, pastas, side dishes, and snacks
- Many restaurant meals (see Appendix A: Ten Tips for Eating Out)
- Most fast foods
- Most pizza, fresh or frozen
- Pre-made "fresh" foods, such as sandwiches, entrées, soups, sides, and snacks
- Pre-seasoned or pre-sauced "ready to cook" foods

Snacks

- Cheese puffs
- Commercial snack "mixes"
- Corn chips
- Frozen snacks
- Jerky and meat sticks (beef, turkey, etc.)
- Most Asian-style chips, nuts, and crackers
- Most commercial trail mixes
- Most granola, energy, protein, and power bars
- Most store-bought smoothies
- Pork rinds
- Potato chips
- Pre-popped or microwave popcorn
- Snack crackers
- Store-bought dips and spreads
- Tortilla chips
- Vegetable chips

Refined Grains

- Instant oatmeal
- Most commercial breakfast cereals, breads, crackers, tortillas, wraps, croutons, and bread crumbs
- Most commercial granola
- Pasta made from white flour
- White flour
- White rice

Prepared Vegetables

- Canned tomatoes, except no salt added
- Canned vegetables, except low-sodium
- Deep-fried vegetables, such as zucchini sticks and tempura
- French fries, home fries, and hash browns
- Frozen vegetables in sauce
- Most commercial vegetable juices
- Pickled, preserved, or brined vegetables
- Vegetables sautéed in butter

Prepared Fruits

- Canned fruit packed in light or heavy syrup
- Frozen fruit packed in syrup
- Most commercial fruit juices

Meats, Poultry, Seafood, and Eggs

- Bacon (pork, poultry, or beef)
- Barbecued or smoked meats, such as ribs and pulled pork
- Beef: brisket, filet mignon/tenderloin, flap, ground (except lean), marrow bones, oxtail, porterhouse, prime rib, rib eye, short ribs, skirt, strip, and T-bone
- Canned meats
- Chicken and turkey: drumsticks, ground (except lean), skin, thighs, and wings
- Deep-fried protein, including chicken, fish, and tofu

- Lamb: breast, all ground, and shoulder
- Many deli meats, such as bologna, chicken roll, corned beef, ham, and pastrami
- Most smoked fish
- Oil-packed canned fish
- Pre-made fish and meat salads
- Pre-seasoned vegetable protein, such as tofu
- Pork: belly, all ground, lard, ribs, and shoulder
- Sausages, such as bratwurst, hot dogs, Italian sausage, pepperoni, and salami

Dairy

- Cream or cheese sauces
- Fried cheeses
- Full-fat sour cream
- Half-and-half
- Hard and semi-firm cheeses
- Heavy or whipping cream
- Whole milk
- Yogurt (even low-fat and nonfat) that is flavored with fruit or other additives

Nuts, Seeds, and Legumes

- Canned legumes, except for low-sodium
- Commercial nut butters, except for "natural" versions that separate into layers in the jar
- Nut butters with added flavorings, such as jelly or chocolate
- Salted nut butters
- Salted, oil-roasted, honey-roasted, smoked, or flavored nuts

Fats

- Butter
- Cottonseed oil

- Palm oil
- Stick margarine and other margarines with partially or fully hydrogenated oils or trans fats
- "Vegetable oil" (a blend of oils that might include bad fats)
- Vegetable shortening

Sweets

- Artificial sweeteners, such as aspartame, saccharine, and sucralose
- Breakfast pastries, such as croissants, Danishes, doughnuts, and sticky buns
- Candy bars
- Candy "truffles"
- Commercial and store-bought baked goods
- Conventional baked goods, such as brownies, cakes, cookies, muffins, and pies
- Conventional cheesecake
- Dessert pastries, such as cannoli, éclairs, and tiramisu
- Fudge
- Fudge or caramel sauces
- Ice cream
- Milk shakes
- Most commercial chocolate bars
- Most store-bought custard, flan, and pudding
- Table sugar

Extras

- Commercial salad dressings, marinades, and sauces
- Full-fat mayonnaise
- Ketchup
- Mustard
- Nondairy creamer
- Packaged gravy, sauce, and seasoning mixes
- Table salt and salt substitutes

TOP TEN DASH DIET FAQS

1. **How soon can I expect to see results?** NIH studies show that the DASH diet starts to lower blood pressure in fourteen days. The DASH diet is also designed to help you lose (if you wish to) one to two pounds per week—the rate most medical professionals consider to be healthful. You might lose even more the first week or two, as your body flushes out the water weight caused by nutritional imbalances such as excess sodium; deficiencies of protein, vitamin B, calcium, magnesium, and potassium; and dehydration.

2. **I thought eggs had a lot of cholesterol. Can I really eat them?** Yes. Eggs are a great source of protein if they are eaten in moderation. All of their cholesterol (185 mg to 210 mg, depending on the size) is in the yolk, so one choice is to eat only the egg white. (You can buy egg whites at the supermarket in a carton; just make sure whatever you buy has no additives.) If you want the yolk, remember that you should limit dietary cholesterol to less than 300 mg per day and to less than 200 mg per day if you have high blood cholesterol. On days when you eat eggs (no more than one per day), cut back on other sources of cholesterol, such as meat and dairy. You may also try low-cholesterol egg substitutes.

3. **I'm lactose intolerant or have a dairy allergy. If I leave dairy products out of my DASH diet, can I still get enough protein and calcium?** Yes. Try lactose-free dairy products or those made with goat's milk. You might be able to tolerate yogurt, cheeses, or even nonfat dairy items. If not, eliminate the dairy and make sure you get enough protein and calcium from other sources, such as dark leafy greens, almonds, and sardines for calcium, and eggs, beans, and nuts for protein.

4. **I have celiac disease or a gluten allergy. How can I adapt to the DASH diet's emphasis on grains?** You know you need to avoid wheat and anything made with wheat, including a wide range of surprising foods, such as soy sauce, gravies, and beer. You also need to stay away from some other grains, such as spelt, barley, rye, and certain oat products. Instead, choose gluten-free whole grains, such as brown rice, buckwheat, and quinoa.

5. **The DASH diet recommends limiting sodium to 1,500 to 2,300 mg per day. Exactly how much is the right amount for me?** For good health, it's best for everyone to keep their sodium intake as low as possible within that range. If you have high blood pressure, you should be eating

1,500 mg or even less. Or, if you're in one of the population groups who are at high risk of developing hypertension, such as people over fifty, African Americans, diabetics, or kidney disease patients, you should also keep to the lower limit.

6. **Can the DASH diet reduce my blood pressure even if I don't make drastic cuts to my sodium intake?** It depends. Losing weight lowers blood pressure, especially if you drop belly fat. Eating plenty of whole grains, fruits, and vegetables and reducing saturated fat and cholesterol in your diet can also lower your blood pressure. Exercise is another effective tool. However, you'll see faster, bigger, and longer-lasting results if you limit sodium in your diet.

7. **Can't I lose weight and get healthy just by cutting calories and taking vitamins or other dietary supplements?** You can certainly lose weight that way, but the DASH diet is more effective for losing weight, keeping it off, and improving your health. The nutrients in healthful food are absorbed more readily than those in supplements, and work together better for weight loss and blood pressure reduction.

8. **Can I use recipes other than the ones in this book?** Yes—and you should! Variety is the spice of a successful diet. It's easy to find delicious, nutritious recipes for meals that follow DASH recommendations or to tweak many other recipes to make them work. If you're comfortable in the kitchen, you can invent your own DASH-friendly dishes. Wherever your recipes come from, just make sure that they use only DASH-recommended ingredients in the amounts laid out in this book. Always remember the correct portion sizes and make sure you get the recommended number of servings of each food group each day.

9. **Do I have to exercise?** It's a very good idea. Exercise reduces blood pressure, burns calories, supports your metabolism, fights fatigue, improves sleep, and boosts overall health. Even moderate exercise like walking can make a big difference, and you can reap the benefits with just thirty minutes of exercise three times a week. You may even divide those thirty minutes into two fifteen-minute or three ten-minute sessions. But you don't have to jump right into running, fitness classes, or bicycling. Start as slowly as you need to, and step it up as your health improves. If your days are crazy busy, take shorter workout breaks when and where you may throughout the day. Five minutes of deep knee bends in your office does a world of good.

10. **How can the DASH diet keep me from gaining back the weight I lose?** Once you adapt to the DASH diet, you're likely to enjoy your new way of eating and how it makes you feel. You'll learn that healthful eating doesn't have to mean deprivation. Even though you'll be eating smaller portions, you won't feel hungry or have as many cravings for salty, sugary, and fatty foods. You'll still be able to indulge a few times a week. And you'll see how fabulous you look. Put that all together, and you're a whole lot less likely to return to bad eating habits than you would be after many other diets.

CHAPTER TWO

How to Use the Meal Plan

Before you start any project, whether it's renovating the bathroom, implementing a business plan, or taking a vacation, your chances of successfully completing it go way up if you start with a clear plan. It's the same with the DASH diet: Planning ahead is essential to make the most of the program.

WHY THE DASH DIET MEAL PLAN WORKS

Well-defined, specific, and realistic daily, weekly, and monthly meal plans make DASH easier and more effective in many ways.

- Developing meal plans solidifies your understanding of DASH guidelines, making it easier to follow them.
- Designing your menus ahead of time helps you establish healthful eating habits and leave unhealthful patterns behind.
- Deciding on your food choices ahead of time makes it more likely that you'll choose the right foods.
- Buying and keeping meal-plan foods on hand ensures that you eat right when you're hungry.
- Setting up a firm meal plan saves you time when you shop for food and helps you avoid temptation at the store.
- Knowing what you're going to be eating lets you plan out your shopping to save money using coupons and specials and to avoid buying food that will go to waste.
- Having a menu plan enables you to prepare food in advance and pre-portion it into storage containers.
- Anticipating the delicious meals that await you prepares you for satisfaction.

MAKE THE MOST OF YOUR MEAL PLAN

Meal planning is an unbeatable opportunity to customize the DASH diet to your weight and health goals, dietary needs, culinary tastes, and lifestyle. There's a lot of flexibility in what you eat within the basic DASH framework:

- A substantial breakfast within an hour of getting up
- A generous lunch
- A small snack about two hours before dinner
- A light dinner no less than three hours before bedtime

Because it emphasizes eating healthful food over counting calories, DASH doesn't require that each of the meals deliver a particular number of calories. Nor must you eat specific foods at specific meals, though it's best to get some protein and complex carbohydrates at each meal. It's fine if you feel like eating vegetables for breakfast and eggs for dinner, as long as you eat your total required servings from each food group.

When planning the menu for the day, be sure to include:

- 7–8 servings of whole grains
- 4–5 servings of vegetables
- 4–5 servings of fruits
- 2–3 servings of nonfat or low-fat dairy products
- No more than 2 servings total of lean meats, poultry, seafood, and eggs
- No more than 2 servings of fats and oils

Over the course of a week, work in:

- 4–5 servings of nuts, seeds, and legumes
- No more than 2 servings total of sweets and added sugars

When it comes to meal size, the United States suffers from "portion distortion." Bombarded with super-size, jumbo, family-size, extra-value, mega, and all-you-can-eat dining options, Americans have lost track of how big a healthful serving of food should be. When making your DASH meal plan, refer to the DASH Diet Food Guidelines chart in Chapter One for examples of correct serving sizes.

LEARN TO READ FOOD LABELS

The DASH eating plan focuses on fresh vegetables, fruits, and proteins, which you buy raw and prepare yourself. You can purchase many of the grains, nuts, seeds, and legumes from bulk bins, without any added ingredients. But any time you buy packaged food—even items labeled "natural," "organic," "nonfat," "low-sodium," "no sugar added," and the like—it's crucial to read the ingredients list and the Nutrition Facts label.

Inspect the ingredients list and reject any food that's heavy on refined grains, sugar, salt, or anything on the DASH Foods to Avoid list in Chapter One. Then look at the size of the print on the ingredients label. If it's too small to read, that's a clue that there might be a whole lot of ingredients in the product. More ingredients often means more stuff that's bad for you, such as artificial flavors, sweeteners, and colors or a whole laboratory's worth of emulsifiers, flavor enhancers (such as monosodium glutamate), preservatives, stabilizers, and thickeners. Some of the mystery matter might include hidden sugars, high-fructose corn syrup, bad fats, or sodium. If you see a lot of ingredients that you can't pronounce or decipher, it's a good idea to put the package back on the shelf.

The government-mandated Nutrition Facts label, that information box printed on every packaged food product in the store, is a treasure trove of DASH data. It doesn't tell you everything you'd like to know, but it's still a valuable tool. Take a look at the example here.

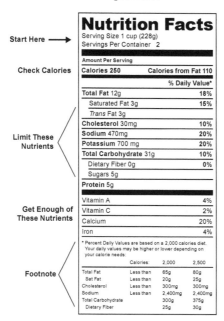

The "serving size" and "servings per container" at the top of the label give you an understanding of how much food is actually in the package. The "calories" line indicates how many calories and fat-based calories are in *one* serving (based on the stated serving size). Below that, the lines for nutrients, from "total fat" down to "protein," give the weight (in grams) of each nutrient that's contained in a single serving.

Another measurement, the "percent daily value," is given for each of the nutrients as well as for some vitamins and minerals. Percent daily value is based on government recommendations for how much of a given substance a 2,000-calorie-per-day diet should include. For instance, the 15 percent figure for saturated fat in the example label means one serving contains 15 percent of the saturated fat you should eat in a 2,000-calorie day. If a vitamin or mineral doesn't appear in the Nutrition Facts label, the food isn't a significant source of the nutrient. The basic rule is that a food is considered low in any nutrients with a daily value of 5 percent or less and high in those with a daily value of 20 percent or more.

Except for the milligrams of sodium, the numbers on the Nutrition Facts label don't translate directly into DASH diet guidelines. Nevertheless, they're good benchmarks for evaluating if a packaged food makes sense for your weight-loss regime. If you're trying to reduce your blood pressure, though, that sodium measurement is golden information.

SHOPPING TIPS

The first rule of healthful shopping is "plan ahead." That's exactly what the DASH diet meal plan helps you do. The second rule is "read the labels." If you've read the preceding Learn to Read Food Labels section, you've got that one squared away. Here are a few more tips.

- Focus your shopping on the perimeter of the supermarket. That's usually where you'll find fresh foods such as vegetables, fruits, meat, poultry, fish, and dairy.
- Spend a minimum amount of time in your supermarket's center aisles, where the processed, packaged, and junk foods are. Brave those aisles

only to pick up pantry items like oatmeal, whole-wheat pasta, olive oil, and spices.

- Look for the bulk section of the store, where you may scoop what you want out of bins containing grains, nuts, seeds, dried legumes, and flours. Except for the salted nuts, granolas, pastas, and snack items, bulk items are simple, single-ingredient products without undesirable ingredients.
- Compare similar items—say, multigrain breads—and choose the one with the fewest number of ingredients (unless those ingredients aren't "real").
- If they're available and you can afford them, choose organic ingredients, and meat, dairy, and eggs that are free of antibiotics, growth hormones, and steroids.
- For the freshest food, choose items grown locally, if possible. Farmers' markets and farm stands are great for this. If you don't have local options, look for food grown nearer rather than farther away. Think Texas instead of Thailand.

STOCK YOUR PANTRY

Day to day and week to week on the DASH diet, you'll be using certain ingredients again and again. Many of them will be fresh items such as leafy greens, chicken breasts, or yogurt, but many others will be pantry items with a long shelf life. You'll be using some pantry items only occasionally, so buy them as needed, but make your life easier by always keeping these ingredients on hand.

- Additives: arrowroot powder, baking powder, baking soda
- Beverages: club soda (seltzer), dried herbal teas, unsweetened non-dairy milks (unsweetened almond, hemp, quinoa, rice, or soy)
- Canned tomatoes, no salt added
- Condiments: apple cider vinegar, balsamic vinegar, hot sauce
- Dried herbs: basil, bay leaves, marjoram, oregano, parsley, rosemary, sage, tarragon, thyme
- Flours: brown rice, buckwheat, medium-grind stone-ground cornmeal, whole-wheat
- Legumes (low-sodium, if canned): black beans, chickpeas (garbanzo beans), lentils, split peas, white beans (cannellini, great northern, navy)
- Nut and seed butters, unsalted: almond, peanut, tahini (sesame)

- Nuts (unsalted raw or dry-roasted): almonds, peanuts, pine nuts (pignoli), walnuts
- Oils: canola, extra-virgin olive, sesame
- Pastas: brown rice, quinoa, whole-wheat
- Proteins: unsweetened powders (egg, hemp, pea, soy, whey)
- Seeds (unsalted raw or dry-roasted): flax, pumpkin (pepita), sesame, sunflower
- Spices: black peppercorns, cayenne, chili powder, cinnamon, cocoa powder (unsweetened), coriander, crushed red pepper flakes, cumin, curry powder, nutmeg, paprika, pure vanilla extract
- Sweeteners: honey, pure maple syrup
- Whole grains: brown rice, bulgur, quinoa, steel-cut and rolled whole oats, wheat berries, whole-grain barley (not pearled)

BASIC EQUIPMENT

You don't have to go out and buy a bunch of expensive, exotic kitchen equipment to do your DASH cooking. In addition to the basics—pots and pans, knives, whisks, spatulas, mixing bowls, measuring cups, baking dishes, and so on—that you probably have already, these tools can help you make the most of your time in the kitchen.

Recommended

- 8-inch chef's knife, sharp
- Airtight storage containers (various sizes)
- Blender (countertop or immersion style)
- Citrus reamer
- Citrus zester
- Closed-top beverage pitcher or jug
- Food processor
- Kitchen scale
- Parchment paper
- Pepper grinder
- Plastic zip-top bags
- Steamer basket

Nice to Have

- Cast-iron skillet
- Countertop electric mixer
- Electric citrus juicer
- Electric griddle/panini press
- Electric vegetable/fruit juicer
- Slow cooker
- Toaster oven

COOKING TECHNIQUES

Rule number one of the DASH diet is to cut out commercially processed and store-bought prepared foods. When you do so, you'll be doing a lot more cooking. If you're not big on kitchen work, that might seem like a grim prospect. But there are a couple of simple ways to keep your cooking easy and appetizing.

When you bring home the haul from a shopping excursion, do some advance preparation of your fresh ingredients. Look over the week's meal plan to see how the fruits and vegetables should be prepped, and take care of it right then, so that your ingredients are ready to go when it's time to cook. That might mean peeling, coring, seeding, chopping, or grating. Then prepare your meats, poultry, and fish, cutting large pieces into portion sizes, removing any skin from chicken or turkey, and cutting all visible fat off the meat. For any prepped food that will be used in more than one recipe, divide it up accordingly. Refrigerate everything in tightly sealed containers or zip-top bags until you need it.

You can do advance prep for upcoming meals any time you have the opportunity. You can even take the preparations further, depending on what makes sense for the recipes. You might do some initial cooking, such as broiling chicken breasts, you might pre-assemble a casserole so it's ready to pop into the oven, or you might cook a big pot of soup.

Success with the DASH diet depends not only on cooking the right foods but also on cooking them the right way. Fortunately, the most healthful ways of cooking are often the easiest and the tastiest. Clean and simple, these techniques elevate the natural flavors of fresh ingredients, rather than hiding them under fat, salt, and sugar. Use these methods for marvelous results.

- **Baking:** Not just for bread and casseroles, fat-free baking produces pleasing protein, vegetable, and egg dishes.
- **Blanching:** Overcooking vegetables strips them of flavor, color, and nutrients. Enter blanching, a technique in which you boil your vegetables briefly to a crisp-tender texture, then drain them and use them however you like. To stop the hot vegetables from continuing to cook, plunge them into ice water.
- **Boiling:** Put water in a pot with dry grains, dry legumes, or root vegetables and put the pot on the stove over high heat. No fat, lots of flavor.
- **Braising:** A method most often associated with meat and poultry, braising on the stove or in the oven is also good for vegetables. After a sear in a skillet with a small amount of fat, the food cooks in a covered pot, slowly and at a low temperature, in liquid such as broth or vegetable juice. The braising liquid is served along with the main ingredient, sometimes reduced into gravy. Braising yields rich, tender, low-fat results, even if you start with tough meat.
- **Broiling:** Your oven's broiler is the hottest tool for indoor cooking. The high heat seals in the juices of meat, poultry, and fish, while allowing any fat to drain through the slots in the cooking surface and into the drip pan.
- **Grilling:** Like broiling, grilling lets fat melt away from your food. But cooking over a fire adds and intensifies flavor. Use the technique for any of your proteins, many of your vegetables, and some of your fruit.
- **Poaching:** Similar to braising, poaching is a quicker way to cook ingredients in liquid. You don't sear the ingredients first, so there's no added fat, and you finish by turning off the heat and leaving the ingredients in the covered pot to continue cooking for several minutes. Poaching is best for delicate ingredients such as chicken, fish, and eggs.
- **Roasting:** A higher-temperature version of baking, roasting uses the dry heat of your oven to seal in and intensify flavor. Vegetables—especially root vegetables—become sweeter, nuts and seeds get nice and toasty, and proteins give up their fats (use a rack in the roasting pan to keep the food out of the fat).
- **Sautéing:** You might think it takes a lot of oil or butter to sauté, but you can get delightful results with this quick stovetop technique using just a little bit of fat or even water or broth. Sautéing is perfect for vegetables—especially onions and leafy greens—whole or cut-up chicken breasts, and fish filets.

- **Searing:** This is a fantastic way to enhance the flavor of meats, poultry, and some seafood. With just a little oil in a hot, hot skillet, you can seal in the juices and create a delicious outer crust. For thicker cuts of meat, fish steaks, and chicken breasts, finish the cooking in the oven.
- **Steaming:** Vegetables and seafood are the stars of the steamer basket, which holds them above a small amount of boiling water in a covered pot. You can add herbs to the water to infuse the food with extra flavor.

FLAVOR TIPS

When you ditch processed foods and start cooking the DASH way, you might at first miss your crunchy, salty fries and creamy, sugary ice cream cones. But stick with it and you'll lose your appetite for overblown seasoning as your taste buds rediscover the delights of pure food.

An average slice of plain cheese pizza has about 550 mg of sodium. A twelve-ounce can of soda hides about ten teaspoons of refined sugar. The typical chain restaurant cheeseburger contains about 25 mg of saturated fat. Americans have become addicted to salty, sweet, fatty foods. Herbs and spices may help you break the habit.

In the meantime, the recipes in this book will show you how to keep your meals exciting. All it takes is a pinch of herbs and spices—among which you have hundreds of choices. Here are some of the readily available standouts.

- **Basil:** Especially when fresh, basil has a heady aroma and a lightly licorice-like flavor that goes especially well with tomatoes, chicken, and fish. It's great in salad dressing, too.
- **Black pepper:** The sharp heat of freshly ground black pepper zings up just about any dish, from soup to steak.
- **Chile pepper:** Your supermarket no doubt carries several varieties of dried hot chiles, such as crushed red pepper flakes, chili powder, cayenne pepper, and tiny Thai chiles. You can fire up almost any savory dish, as well as chocolate, with these hotties.
- **Cinnamon:** Ground or in sticks, cinnamon lends a sweet warmth to fruit, dairy, baked goods, and desserts, not to mention oatmeal.

- **Coriander/cilantro:** The dried seeds of the plant are called coriander and the leaves are called cilantro. Coriander is used whole or crushed in many Mexican and Indian dishes. Cilantro has a refreshing piquancy that matches well with everything from lime to fish.
- **Cumin:** Aromatic and herbaceously peppery, cumin seeds are used both whole and ground. They're a cornerstone of Indian, Middle Eastern, and South American cuisine and work wonders with bean and vegetable dishes and mixed with yogurt.
- **Curry powder:** Most often associated with Indian cuisine, this spice blend may include any combination of coriander, cumin, turmeric, red and black pepper, ginger, fennel seed, cinnamon, clove, mustard seed, and more. Sometimes hot, sometimes almost sweet, it's a wonderful complement to vegetable stews and chicken.
- **Garlic:** The king of flavorings, garlic is a vegetable that's used like an herb to flavor other ingredients. It pairs beautifully with just about any vegetable or protein, particularly in Asian- and Mediterranean-inspired recipes.
- **Ginger:** You can find ginger in both the produce and spice departments of your supermarket. When minced or grated, the gnarled beige fingers of fresh ginger touch Asian-style dishes with sweet heat. Dried ginger powder has a more subdued flavor that's great in curries and sweet baked goods.
- **Marjoram:** Related to oregano, marjoram has a milder, less pungent flavor that works well with mushrooms, eggs, beans, and most proteins.
- **Nutmeg:** A tiny bit of earthy, spicy ground nutmeg goes a long way in both sweet and savory meat- and dairy-based recipes as well as baked items.
- **Onion:** Used both as a vegetable and an herb, onion can be sharp when raw or sweet when cooked. It lends depth to any savory flavor profile, whether in vegetable, protein, bean, or grain dishes.
- **Oregano:** The strong, spicy herb is widely used in Italy and also throughout the Mediterranean. It goes with anything involving tomatoes and is lovely with fish and chicken.
- **Rosemary:** Rosemary has a distinctive piney flavor and aroma that evokes sunny Mediterranean lands. It's an excellent complement to meat and poultry and is a wonderful flavoring for olive oil.
- **Sage:** Somewhat peppery and minty, sage is a familiar addition to roasted, baked, and grilled poultry. Its big flavor lends depth to many bold, rich dishes.

- **Tarragon:** Tasting like mild, sweet licorice, tarragon is much used in French cuisine. It pairs well with fish, chicken, and eggs and makes a lovely infusion with vinegar.
- **Thyme:** Another essential flavor in French cooking, thyme is also a major ingredient in Middle Eastern cuisine. Its tiny leaves taste a bit minty and lemony, with the lemony component amplified in a delicious variety called lemon thyme. Thyme is a great addition to all kinds of recipes, especially soups, sauces, and salad dressings.

TEN STEPS TO SUCCESS WITH THE DASH DIET MEAL PLAN

Making meal plans is one key to succeeding with the DASH diet. But how do you make the most of your meal planning; how do you make it a success? Changing the way you eat will most likely be a challenge at first, especially if you've been a fan of super-size fries, extra-large pizzas, and giant sodas. But DASH gives you so many tasty foods to choose from and so much flexibility in what you eat day to day, that in a week or two it won't feel like a diet at all. These ten steps will help you get on track and stay there.

1. **Plan smart.** Be realistic when laying out your monthly, weekly, and daily meal plans. Don't include meals that are too complicated for your skills, too time-consuming for your schedule, or too awkward to eat away from home.
2. **Plan for enjoyment.** Work out menus that your taste buds will appreciate. Adapt favorite meals, if possible, and keep using healthful ingredients you know and like. Leave out ingredients or dishes you don't like. Don't force yourself to make rapid, radical changes in your eating habits.
3. **Shop well.** Use your meal plans to write a shopping list that includes only the ingredients of the dishes in your meal plan, and bring it to the store with you. Don't deviate from the list while you're shopping. (Also take advantage of the Shopping Tips in this chapter.)
4. **Eliminate distractions.** Ditch anything in your house, office, or car that isn't part of your meal plan. Search your cupboards, refrigerator, freezer, pantry, hiding places, desk drawers, and glove compartment for junk food and processed food, and get rid of it. Throw it out or give it away. (Refer to the Foods to Avoid list in Chapter One for recommendations.)

5. **Include your family.** If you live with family, friends, or roommates, explain your meal plan and encourage them to eat what you eat. Turning them on to healthful eating makes it easier to clear your home of bad food, and you won't end up shopping for or cooking two (or more) menus for every meal.

6. **Be prepared.** Avoid temptation by making it easy to follow your plan. Stock your pantry and refrigerator with meal plan items that will be ready when you are. Keep prepped snacks, ready-to-use ingredients, and precooked meals on hand. (The Cooking Techniques section in this chapter has some suggestions.)

7. **Plan your schedule as well as your menu.** Set up an eating plan with a preset daily timetable so you won't miss meals. Knowing when you're eating your next meal makes it easier to resist temptation between meals, and keeping regular mealtimes helps your body adjust to the DASH diet.

8. **Plan for dining out.** It's easiest to follow the DASH guidelines if you cook your own food, but if you like to dine out, work restaurant meals into your plan. For example, allot two lunches or one dinner per week to dining out. If your meal plan allows for the occasional "cheat," consider making it part of your restaurant meal. See Appendix A: Ten Tips for Dining Out for more strategies.

9. **Plan for special occasions.** Whether it's Thanksgiving dinner with the family or brunch with friends, put it on your DASH calendar as far ahead of time as you can. If you're doing the entertaining, create an appropriately festive menu with DASH-friendly dishes. If you're a guest, do your best to choose the most healthful options and eat the correct portions (you don't have to bring your own food). Don't worry about perfection; just pay attention. As with restaurant dining, if your meal plan allows for off-DASH indulgence, a special occasion is the perfect time to treat yourself.

10. **Keep track.** Buy a notebook or a smartphone app and keep a journal of what and when you eat each day. Be accurate by writing your notes as soon as you eat, and be honest. After all, you're doing the DASH diet *for you*. Recording what you eat makes you more mindful of your diet, and comparing it to your meal plan enables you to get back on track when you've lost your focus. Keep your eye on the prize!

PART TWO

Putting the DASH Diet Meal Plan into Action

f you fail to plan, you plan to fail." When it comes to improving the way you eat, this old adage couldn't be more apt. Planning your shopping and eating strategies ahead of time takes the guesswork and distractions out of your health-improvement program, tremendously increasing your chances of success.

The developers of this diet recommend that you make the transition gradually, adopting different parts of the eating plan week by week, rather than trying to do it all in a few days. The daily menu plans in the next four chapters will guide you through the first four weeks of your DASH transformation. With three meals and a snack included in each day's plan, plus dessert, your food choices, sodium consumption, and calorie intake are all laid out for you.

If you want to follow these plans exactly, great! Your path to a better diet is clearly mapped out for you, and you won't have to figure out a thing. If you prefer to tinker and adjust the plans to suit your own tastes and lifestyle, great! Just put the basic DASH guidelines into action, and you'll be able to create a delicious, healthful diet that's easy for you to follow.

The four-week DASH diet meal plan laid out here delivers up to 2,000 calories and 1,600 mg of sodium a day. Some days come in lower than that, which means you get to eat more of the good stuff! Each week's program encompasses a wide variety of tasty foods. The recipes in Part Three include everything except the snacks, but no two days in the plan have the same menu.

All the ingredients you'll need are itemized in weekly shopping lists for you to take to the supermarket. Plan-ahead preparation suggestions point out ways to get your ingredients ready in advance, at your convenience, for easier, quicker cooking—or *no* cooking—at mealtime. And throughout, tips for buying food, using ingredients, cooking dishes, managing nutrition, living well, and handling challenges smooth your path to success.

Week One

The DASH diet recommends making gradual changes to one's diet and lifestyle in order to lower blood pressure. Rather than switching from one's normal diet to the DASH diet all at once, [you] are encouraged to slowly adopt and adjust to different parts of the eating plan over a period of time.

—Wellness.com, "DASH Diet"

WEEK ONE MEAL PLAN

Day One

Total sodium: 1,448 mg

Breakfast
Peanut Butter and Banana Smoothie
Sodium per serving: 200 mg
Lunch
Pepper Steak Salad
Sodium per serving: 584 mg
Snack
1 (1-ounce) granola bar
Sodium per serving: 75 mg

Dinner

Three-Bean Chili

Sodium per serving: 469 mg

Zesty Quinoa

Sodium per serving: 103 mg

Dessert

Strawberry-Banana Frozen Yogurt

Sodium per serving: 17 mg

Daily Tip: A few basic kitchen tools may help you minimize the fat in your cooking. Buy a nonstick skillet and saucepan so you use less oil. Put a rack in the baking dish when you roast meat or poultry to keep them out of the fatty drippings. Use your broiler or outdoor grill, so melted fat trickles away. An indoor electric grill may do the trick, too.

Day Two

Total sodium: 1,106 mg

Breakfast

Honey-Walnut Fruit Salad

Sodium per serving: 3 mg

Lunch

Chicken Quesadillas with Pico de Gallo

Sodium per serving: 309 mg

Snack

1 large hard-boiled egg

Sodium per serving: 62 mg

Dinner

Orange-Flavored Beef with Stir-Fried Vegetables

Sodium per serving: 390 mg

Brown Rice Pilaf

Sodium per serving: 178 mg

Dessert

Death by Chocolate Cupcakes

Sodium per serving: 164 mg

Daily Tip: Cut back on bad fats by using margarine instead of butter when you're baking. Go for soft tub margarine rather than the firmer stick margarine, which contains cholesterol-sabotaging trans fat. But not all tub margarines are created equal. Pick the ones labeled "0 grams trans fat" and avoid the ones with "hydrogenated" or "partially hydrogenated" oils in the list of ingredients.

Day Three

Total sodium: 1,407 mg

Breakfast
Apple-Cinnamon Oatmeal
Sodium per serving: 293 mg

Lunch
Mini English Muffin Pizzas
Sodium per serving: 365 mg

Snack
¼ cup garlic-dill yogurt with ¼ medium cucumber
Sodium per serving: 24 mg

Dinner
Baked BBQ Chicken
Sodium per serving: 497 mg
Jalapeño Cornbread
Sodium per serving: 103 mg

Dessert
The Original Flan
Sodium per serving: 125 mg

Daily Tip: Even if you're an experienced cook who's confident in the kitchen, measure all your ingredients for at least your first week on the DASH plan. You might be surprised how inaccurate your "eyeball" is.

Day Four

Total sodium: 1,512 mg

Breakfast
Herbed Asparagus and Balsamic Onion Frittata
Sodium per serving: 396 mg
Lunch
Tuna-Apple Salad Sandwiches
Sodium per serving: 231
Snack
2 cups homemade lemon-garlic kale chips
Sodium per serving: 242 mg
Dinner
Green Lasagna
Sodium per serving: 310 mg
Parmesan-Crusted Cauliflower
Sodium per serving: 209 mg
Dessert
Heavenly Apple Crisp
Sodium per serving: 124 mg

Daily Tip: If you use dried herbs instead of fresh, measure out one unit (teaspoon, tablespoon, etc.) of dried to three units of fresh. Unlike fresh herbs, which are best when added toward the end of the cooking process, dried herbs should be added early in the game. Their flavors really pop with at least thirty minutes of cooking.

Day Five

Total sodium: 1,254 mg

Breakfast
Blueberry and Oat Pancakes
Sodium per serving: 288 mg
Lunch
Turkey Noodle Soup
Sodium per serving: 434 mg

Snack

¼ cup hummus with 12 baby carrots

Sodium per serving: 148 mg

Dinner

Creamy Sole with Grapes

Sodium per serving: 193 mg

Aromatic Almond Couscous

Sodium per serving: 99 mg

Dessert

Chocolate–Sweet Potato Pudding

Sodium per serving: 92 mg

> **Daily Tip:** Eating fish that's high in omega-3 fatty acids, which fall into the category of polyunsaturated fat, may help bring your blood pressure down and lower your risk of having a heart attack. Some fish, such as tuna, salmon, trout, mackerel, and herring, are especially rich in omega-3s.

Day Six

Total sodium: 1,437 mg

Breakfast

Tropical Strawberry Shake

Sodium per serving: 164 mg

Lunch

Southwestern Quinoa–Black Bean Salad

Sodium per serving: 315 mg

Snack

¼ cup light ricotta cheese with 1 tablespoon walnuts and 1 teaspoon honey

Sodium per serving: 56 mg

Dinner

Chicken-Asparagus Penne

Sodium per serving: 476 mg

Tuscan Kale Salad Massaged with Roasted Garlic

Sodium per serving: 244 mg

Dessert
Carrot-Raisin-Oatmeal Cookies
Sodium per serving: 182 mg

· ·

Daily Tip: A serving of pasta consists of one cup of cooked noodles. But of course, not all noodles are shaped the same, so a cup of cooked noodles can vary in weight. To be sure, for a one-cup yield, start with 2 ounces of dry pasta per serving.

· ·

Day Seven

Total sodium: 1,478 mg

Breakfast
Red, White, and Blue Parfait
Sodium per serving: 62 mg

Lunch
Traditional Beef Stew
Sodium per serving: 607 mg

Snack
⅔ cup frozen banana slices with 1 tablespoon dark chocolate chips
Sodium per serving: 1 mg

Dinner
Crispy Thanksgiving Turkey Fillets
Sodium per serving: 510 mg

Cinnamon-Roasted Glazed Carrots
Sodium per serving: 124 mg

Dessert
Frozen Chocolate–Peanut Butter Pudding Squares
Sodium per serving: 174 mg

· ·

Daily Tip: Generally, the deeper the color of a vegetable or fruit, the higher its vitamin and mineral content. That's why dark, leafy greens are a DASH go-to, as well as bell peppers, carrots, and berries.

· ·

ADDITIONAL TIPS FOR WEEK ONE

- *When* you eat is just as important as *what* you eat. Plan your meal and snack schedule to keep your metabolism fueled and firing. If your body knows that food is on the way soon, it won't slow down to save calories—and store them as fat. A hearty breakfast wakes up your metabolism to burn hot, setting the pace for the day. Eat a sizeable lunch, a small afternoon snack, and a light dinner, and don't eat within three hours of bedtime.
- Packaged foods, even items that you don't think of as salty, may contain a lot of sodium. Carefully read the Nutrition Facts label and the ingredients list. The word *salt* will raise a red flag, of course, but also look out for terms such as *soda, baking soda, sodium bicarbonate, monosodium glutamate (MSG), sodium nitrate, sodium citrate,* and *sodium benzoate.* It's all sodium!
- You're more likely to stick with your new eating habits if your palate is excited. Explore new flavors or combine known ones in new ways. Try your hand at cooking unfamiliar cuisines, or change up your favorite meals by switching the same old side dish for a new one. Keep your plate colorful with a variety of vegetables and fruits.
- The DASH guidelines don't demand that you give up your favorite foods. If you love your guilty pleasures, save them for special occasions and allow yourself a small portion. But don't keep those foods in your home, office, or car.
- Scientists have discovered that salt is an acquired taste. That means you can "un-acquire" your sodium cravings. You might miss salt at first, but before long you'll rediscover the wonderful, natural flavors that have been hiding behind your salt shaker.

WEEK ONE SHOPPING LIST

Pantry Items

- Arrowroot powder
- Baking powder
- Baking soda
- Basil, dried
- Black peppercorns
- Chili powder
- Cinnamon, ground
- Cocoa powder, unsweetened
- Coriander, ground
- Cornstarch
- Cumin, ground
- Ginger, ground
- Honey
- Maple syrup, pure
- Marjoram, dried
- Mustard, dry
- Oil, canola
- Oil, extra-virgin olive
- Oregano, dried
- Paprika
- Red pepper flakes, crushed (optional)
- Rosemary, dried
- Sage, dried
- Salt
- Tarragon, dried
- Thyme, dried
- Vanilla extract, pure
- Vinegar, balsamic
- Vinegar, cider
- Vinegar, red wine

Produce

- Apples, medium (9)
- Arugula (1 pound)
- Asparagus (3 bunches, about 3 pounds)
- Bananas (6)
- Bell peppers, green (2)
- Bell peppers, red (3)
- Bell pepper, yellow (1)
- Blueberries (1½ pounds)
- Broccoli, small heads (2)
- Carrots (20)
- Carrots, baby (12)
- Cauliflower head (1)
- Celery (1 bunch)
- Cherries (8 ounces)
- Chives, fresh (1 bunch)
- Cilantro, fresh (1 bunch)
- Dill, fresh (1 bunch)
- Garlic (3 heads)
- Ginger, fresh (1 ounce)
- Grapes, seedless green (12 ounces)
- Jalapeño peppers (4)
- Kale, curly (1 bunch)
- Kale, Tuscan (4 bunches)
- Lemons (7)
- Lettuce, salad greens (8 ounces)
- Limes (3)

- Mango (1)
- Mushrooms, button or cremini (3 ounces)
- Mushrooms, shiitake (2 ounces)
- Nectarine (1)
- Onion, red (4)
- Onions, white or yellow (9)
- Orange (1)
- Parsley, fresh (1 bunch)
- Potato, white (1)
- Potatoes, sweet (2)
- Raspberries (8 ounces)
- Sage, fresh (1 bunch)
- Scallions (6)
- Strawberries (1 pound)
- Tarragon, fresh (1 bunch)
- Thyme, fresh (1 bunch)
- Tomatoes, cherry (8 ounces)
- Tomatoes (8)
- Zucchini (1)

Protein

- Chicken breasts, boneless, skinless (nine, 3-ounce)
- Chicken drumsticks (two, 4-ounce)
- Chicken thighs, boneless, skinless (two, 3-ounce)
- Sole fillets (four, 3-ounce)
- Steak, flank (12 ounces)
- Steak, top round (1 pound)
- Steak, top sirloin (8 ounces)
- Tuna, low-sodium chunk light in water (two, 6-ounce cans)
- Turkey, skinless breast fillets (four, 3-ounce)
- Turkey, whole, small (1)

Dairy

- Buttermilk, 1 percent (1 pint)
- Cheese, mozzarella, part-skim, shredded (5 ounces)
- Cheese, Parmesan, grated (3 ounces)
- Cheese, pepper Jack, shredded (2 ounces)
- Cheese, ricotta, light (4 ounces)
- Cottage cheese, low-sodium nonfat (12 ounces)
- Margarine, soft tub (4 ounces)
- Milk, 1 percent (1 pint plus 8 ounces)
- Milk, skim (1 quart plus 1 pint)
- Yogurt, nonfat plain Greek (1 quart)

Canned and Bottled Foods

- Applesauce, unsweetened (4 ounces)
- Beans, black, low-sodium (two, 15-ounce cans)

- Beans, pinto, low-sodium (15-ounce can)
- Beans, red kidney, low-sodium (15-ounce can)
- Broth, beef, low-sodium (8 ounces)
- Broth, chicken, low-sodium (1 pint plus 4 ounces)
- Chickpeas, low-sodium (15-ounce can)
- Hoisin sauce (3 ounces)
- Hot sauce (1 ounce)
- Peanut butter, unsalted natural (2½ ounces)
- Pineapple, crushed in juice (two, 15-ounce cans)
- Soy sauce, low-sodium (4 ounces)
- Tahini (1 ounce)
- Tomato paste, no salt added (6-ounce can)
- Tomato sauce, no salt added (three, 14.5-ounce cans)
- Tomatoes, diced, no salt added (14.5-ounce can)
- Tomatoes, diced, no salt added (28-ounce can)
- Worcestershire sauce (1 ounce)

Dry Foods

- Almonds, slivered (4 ounces)
- Bread crumbs, whole-wheat, no salt added (4 ounces)
- Buttermilk powder (2 ounces)
- Cornmeal (7 ounces)
- Couscous, whole-wheat instant (7 ounces)
- Cranberries, dried unsweetened (4 ounces)
- Flour, unbleached all-purpose (8 ounces)
- Flour, whole-wheat (6 ounces)
- Flour, whole-wheat pastry (3 ounces)
- Hazelnuts, unsalted (3 ounces)
- Instant espresso powder (1 teaspoon)
- Lasagna noodles, whole-wheat, dry (12 ounces)
- Milk powder, nonfat (2 ounces)
- Oats, rolled (1 pound)
- Oats, steel-cut (9 ounces)
- Pasta shapes, tiny whole-wheat, dry (8 ounces)
- Penne, whole-wheat, dry (8 ounces)
- Quinoa, dry (11 ounces)
- Raisins (5 ounces)
- Raisins, golden (4 ounces)
- Rice, brown, dry (7 ounces)
- Sugar, confectioners' (1 ounce)
- Sugar, dark brown (2 ounces)
- Sugar, light brown (1 pound)
- Sugar, white (5 ounces)
- Walnuts (3 ounces)

Refrigerated and Frozen Foods

- Eggs (20)
- Banana, frozen (1)
- Strawberries, frozen (10 ounces)

Other

- Almond milk, unsweetened (4 ounces)
- Chocolate chips, dark (½ ounce)
- Coffee, black (6 ounces)
- Cornbread (see Chapter 9) (4-by-4-inch square)
- English muffins, whole-wheat (4)
- Graham crackers (5-ounce package)
- Granola bar (1 ounce)
- Pita pockets, whole-wheat (2)
- Protein powder (1 ounce)
- Sherry, dry (optional) (½ ounce)
- Tortillas, whole-wheat (4)
- White wine, dry (4 ounces)

PLAN-AHEAD PREPARATIONS

This week there are several things you can prepare ahead of time and use throughout the week to make your life easier.

1. **Sliced Vegetables.** Vegetables are everywhere in the DASH diet, and they make great snacks, so save yourself some time during the week by doing your chopping ahead of time in one or two vegetable prep sessions. Vegetables that stand up well to pre-slicing include bell peppers, broccoli, carrots, cauliflower, celery, mushrooms, onions, squash, and sweet potatoes. Just pop them into plastic zip-top bag or sealed containers and put them in the fridge until you're ready to use them.

2. **Chopped Greens.** The DASH plan recommends that you eat lots and lots of leafy greens. You can chop many of these in advance during your weekly or semi-weekly prep sessions. Greens that hold up well to pre-chopping include cabbage, kale, and spinach. Once you prep them, put the greens in a plastic zip-top bag with a paper towel to absorb excess moisture, roll up the bag to squeeze out the air (don't squish the veggies), zip it up, and refrigerate the greens until you're ready to use them.

3. **Breakfasts.** You can make the filling for the Herbed Asparagus and Balsamic Onion Frittata a day in advance and store it in the fridge.

4. **Lunches.** You can make any of the following a day or two in advance: Southwestern Quinoa–Black Bean Salad, Traditional Beef Stew, and Turkey Noodle Soup; the protein portions of the Pepper Steak Salad and Tuna-Apple Salad Sandwiches; and the pico de gallo for the Chicken Quesadillas. Allow hot dishes to cool completely before you put them in the fridge in sealed containers or plastic zip-top bags.

5. **Side Dishes.** You can make any of the following a day in advance: Aromatic Almond Couscous, Brown Rice Pilaf, and Cinnamon-Roasted Glazed Carrots. Allow them to cool completely before you put them in the fridge in sealed containers or plastic zip-top bags.

6. **Dinners.** You can make any of the following a day in advance: Baked BBQ Chicken with Jalapeño Cornbread, Green Lasagna with Parmesan-Crusted Cauliflower, and Three-Bean Chili with Zesty Quinoa. Allow everything to cool completely before you put them in the fridge in sealed containers or plastic zip-top bags.

7. **Desserts.** You can make any of the desserts a day or two in advance and store them in the fridge or freezer.

CHAPTER FOUR

Week Two

People who ate the DASH diet for eight weeks during the study reported feeling better at the end than before starting the diet. Their quality of life improved.... The fact that participants didn't report feeling the same or worse is ... from the perspective of nutritional scientists, a "big deal." Thus, the DASH diet can actually make you feel better.

—Thomas J. Moore, Laura Svetkey, Pao-Hwo Lin, Nieri Karania, and Mark Jenkins, *The DASH Diet for Hypertension*

WEEK TWO MEAL PLAN

Day One

Total sodium: 1,400 mg

Breakfast
Pecan and Sunflower Seed Granola
Sodium per serving: 150 mg
Lunch
Chicken-Lettuce Wraps with Spicy Soy Sauce
Sodium per serving: 297 mg
Snack
¼ cup guacamole with ½ medium whole-wheat tortilla
Sodium per serving: 179 mg

Dinner

Spaghetti with Meat Sauce

Sodium per serving: 440 mg

Spanish-Style Sautéed Baby Spinach

Sodium per serving: 180 mg

Dessert

Fudgy Cookies

Sodium per serving: 154 mg

· ·

Daily Tip: Contrary to what you may have heard, whole-wheat flour works just fine for baking in most recipes. You may generally substitute whole-wheat flour for half the white flour without changing the flavor or texture too much—remember, you don't have to give up white flour completely. Of course, there are exceptions to the whole-wheat rule: Angel food cake, anyone?

· ·

Day Two

Total sodium: 1,575 mg

Breakfast

Apple-Cinnamon Oatmeal

Sodium per serving: 293 mg

Lunch

Creamy Butternut-Apple Soup

Sodium per serving: 366 mg

Snack

16 unsalted raw or dry-roasted cashews, pistachios, or walnuts

Sodium per serving: 0 mg

Dinner

Teriyaki Salmon Stir-Fry

Sodium per serving: 389 mg

Asian Noodles

Sodium per serving: 282 mg

Dessert
Righteous Pumpkin Pie
Sodium per serving: 245 mg

Daily Tip: When you buy fruit and vegetables, keep fiber in mind. Some especially good sources of fiber are artichokes, fresh peas, broccoli, raspberries, oranges, and bananas.

Day Three

Total sodium: 1,487 mg

Breakfast
Apricot-Orange Bread
Sodium per serving: 228 mg

Lunch
Swanky Steak Sandwich
Sodium per serving: 391 mg

Snack
1 medium celery stalk with 1 tablespoon unsalted natural peanut butter
Sodium per serving: 150 mg

Dinner
Comforting Mac and Cheese
Sodium per serving: 192 mg
Lima Beans with Spinach
Sodium per serving: 362 mg

Dessert
Death by Chocolate Cupcakes
Sodium per serving: 164 mg

Daily Tip: A delicious way to cut bad fat and add fiber when you're baking is to use applesauce and canola oil in place of butter. Use a mix of equal parts canola oil and applesauce.

Day Four

Total sodium: 1,253 mg

Breakfast
Peanut Butter and Banana Smoothie
Sodium per serving: 200 mg
Lunch
Hearty Pasta Salad
Sodium per serving: 370 mg
Snack
2 tablespoons homemade whipped cream cheese–sundried tomato spread on
1 (1-ounce) whole-wheat matzo
Sodium per serving: 149 mg
Dinner
Pork Scaloppini with Apple-Raisin Compote
Sodium per serving: 200 mg
Pilaf Parmesan
Sodium per serving: 317 mg
Dessert
Strawberry-Banana Frozen Yogurt
Sodium per serving: 17 mg

Daily Tip: Buying grain such as brown rice from the bulk bins at your supermarket is a great way to save money. Worried that without the box, you won't have cooking directions? No problem. Just follow the one-two-three rule: One cup of dry rice cooked in two cups of water makes three cups of cooked rice.

Day Five

Total sodium: 1,446 mg

Breakfast
Honey-Walnut Fruit Salad
Sodium per serving: 3 mg

Lunch
Fish Tacos
Sodium per serving: 395 mg
Snack
¼ cup chocolate sorbet with 1 tablespoon chopped salted peanuts
Sodium per serving: 65 mg
Dinner
Beef Stroganoff
Sodium per serving: 538 mg
Lemony Roasted Broccoli
Sodium per serving: 320 mg
Dessert
The Original Flan
Sodium per serving: 125 mg

Daily Tip: Not only are low-fat poultry and meat better for your heart, but they're also easier on your digestion. Think of that heavy, sluggish feeling you get after you've downed half a rack of ribs, a big hamburger, or a plate of fried chicken wings.

Day Six

Total sodium: 1,522 mg

Breakfast
Mediterranean Spinach Omelet
Sodium per serving: 441 mg
Lunch
Chicken-Grape Salad Sandwiches
Sodium per serving: 350 mg
Snack
1 ounce (8 small squares) graham crackers
Sodium per serving: 175 mg

Dinner

Beef Tenderloin Mole

Sodium per serving: 226 mg

Black Bean Confetti Salad

Sodium per serving: 176 mg

Dessert

Fudgy Cookies

Sodium per serving: 154 mg

- -

Daily Tip: Believe it or not, you're less likely to hurt yourself in the kitchen with a sharp knife than with a dull one. When you use a dull knife, you have to press down harder to make a cut, so the knife can easily slip or jump into your thumb or palm. A sharp knife slices easily through your food—not through you!

- -

Day Seven

Total sodium: 1,397 mg

Breakfast

Herbed Asparagus and Balsamic Onion Frittata

Sodium per serving: 396 mg

Lunch

Creamy Butternut-Apple Soup

Sodium per serving: 366 mg

Snack

1 ounce dark chocolate

Sodium per serving: 2 mg

Dinner

Oven-Fried Catfish

Sodium per serving: 273 mg

Perfect Coleslaw

Sodium per serving: 236 mg

Dessert

Heavenly Apple Crisp

Sodium per serving: 124 mg

Daily Tip: Certain herbs are far better fresh than dried, among them basil, parsley, cilantro, and dill. Make them last by treating them like flowers: Trim off their ends and put their stems in a container with a little water. Change the water daily to keep it fresh.

ADDITIONAL TIPS FOR WEEK TWO

- Instead of buying cooking oil spray, which may contain flavorings, propellants, and inferior-quality oil, put your extra-virgin olive oil in a spray bottle. You'll have even better control of the calories, fat, and chemicals that go into your cooking.
- Cooking with produce that's in season will give you tastier results. Seasonal fruit and vegetables stay on the stem longer and travel less than produce shipped in from far away, giving them fuller, more intense flavor. And because it's in season, it costs less.
- Drinking too much alcohol can be bad for your heart. Booze raises your blood pressure, damages your heart muscles, and makes you more likely to die if you have a heart attack.
- A handy way to measure your portions is to use your hand. A serving of protein is the size of your palm, a serving of grains is the size of your fist, a serving of vegetables or fruit is the size of two fists, and a serving of fat is the size of your thumb.
- If you're thinking of eating, think twice. Is your stomach growling and hollow? Are you having an emotional or mental craving? Either way, wait fifteen minutes before you eat. Drink a glass of water, put in a load of laundry, brush your teeth. Likely as not, the feeling will pass.

WEEK TWO SHOPPING LIST

Pantry Items

- Allspice, ground
- Baking powder
- Baking soda
- Basil, dried
- Black peppercorns
- Cayenne pepper, ground (optional)
- Celery seeds
- Chili powder

- Cinnamon, ground
- Cocoa powder, unsweetened
- Coriander, ground
- Cumin, ground
- Ginger, ground
- Honey
- Mirin
- Mustard, dry
- Nutmeg, ground
- Oil, canola
- Oil, extra-virgin
- Oil, sesame
- Oregano, dried
- Red pepper flakes, crushed
- Salt
- Vanilla extract, pure
- Vinegar, balsamic
- Vinegar, cider
- Vinegar, rice
- Vinegar, white wine

Produce

- Apples, medium (14)
- Asparagus (1 bunch, about 1 pound)
- Avocado (1)
- Bananas (6)
- Basil, fresh (1 bunch)
- Bell peppers, red (3)
- Bell peppers, yellow (2)
- Blueberries (8 ounces)
- Broccoli heads (2)
- Butternut squash (two, 2¼ to 2½ pounds)
- Cabbage, green (1¼ pounds)
- Cabbage, Napa (Asian) or savoy cabbage (8 ounces)
- Cabbage, red (4 ounces)
- Carrots (6)
- Celery (1 bunch)
- Cilantro, fresh (1 bunch)
- Cucumber (1)
- Fennel bulb (1)
- Garlic (3 heads)
- Ginger, fresh (5 ounces)
- Grapes, seedless green (12 ounces)
- Jalapeño peppers (4)
- Lemons (8)
- Lettuce head, Boston or butter (1)
- Lettuce head, romaine (1)
- Lettuce, salad greens (4 ounces)
- Limes (9)
- Mango (1)
- Mung bean sprouts (4 ounces)
- Mushrooms, button or cremini (10 ounces)
- Nectarine (1)
- Onions, red (3)
- Onions, white or yellow (5)
- Orange (1)
- Oregano, fresh (1 bunch)
- Parsley, fresh (1 bunch)
- Peas, snap or snow (6 ounces)
- Scallions (1 bunch)
- Spinach (2¼ pounds)
- Squash, yellow (1)
- Strawberries (10 ounces)
- Tarragon, fresh (1 bunch)
- Tomatoes, cherry (1 pound)
- Zucchini (1)

Protein

- Beef, ground, extra-lean (1 pound)
- Beef, tenderloin roast (1 pound)
- Beef, top round (1 pound)
- Catfish fillets (six, 5-ounce)
- Chicken breasts, boneless, skinless (ten, 3-ounce)
- Pork tenderloin (2-pound package)
- Salmon fillets (eight, 3-ounce)
- Steak, top round (12 ounces)

Dairy

- Buttermilk, 1 percent (4 ounces)
- Cheese, sharp cheddar, low-fat, finely shredded (6 ounces)
- Cheese, feta, reduced-fat, crumbled (1 ounce)
- Cheese, Parmesan, grated (3 ounces)
- Cream cheese, whipped (1 ounce)
- Margarine, soft tub (5 ounces)
- Milk, skim (1 pint plus 8 ounces)
- Yogurt, nonfat plain Greek (1 quart plus 8 ounces)

Canned and Bottled Foods

- Beans, black, low-sodium (15-ounce can)
- Broth, chicken, low-sodium (12 ounces)
- Chickpeas, low-sodium (15-ounce can)
- Dijon mustard (1½ ounces)
- Evaporated milk, nonfat (five, 12-ounce cans)
- Mayonnaise, light (2 ounces)
- Peanut butter, unsalted natural (1 ounce)
- Pineapple, crushed in juice (15-ounce can)
- Pineapple, diced in juice (15-ounce can)
- Pumpkin (15-ounce can)
- Soy sauce, low-sodium (2 ounces)
- Tomatoes, crushed, no salt added (28-ounce can)
- Tomatoes, sundried (½ ounce)
- Worcestershire sauce (½ ounce)

Dry Foods

- Apricots, dried (1 ounce)
- Asian brown rice vermicelli, dry (8 ounces)
- Bread crumbs, panko (2 ounces)
- Bread crumbs, whole-wheat, no salt added (1 ounce)
- Buttermilk powder (1 ounce)

- Coconut flakes, unsweetened (3 ounces)
- Cranberries, dried unsweetened (2 ounces)
- Egg noodles, whole-wheat, dry (12 ounces)
- Flour, unbleached all-purpose (12 ounces)
- Flour, whole-wheat (5 ounces)
- Flour, whole-wheat pastry (9 ounces)
- Graham cracker crumbs (1 ounce)
- Macaroni, whole-wheat, dry (4 ounces)
- Milk powder, nonfat (1 ounce)
- Oats, rolled (1½ pounds)
- Oats, steel-cut (6 ounces)
- Pasta shapes, whole-wheat (8 ounces)
- Peanuts, salted (1 ounce)
- Pecans (12 ounces)
- Pine nuts (pignoli), toasted (2 ounces)
- Raisins (4 ounces)
- Raisins, golden (3 ounces)
- Rice, white, long-grain, dry (7 ounces)
- Sesame seeds (1 ounce)
- Spaghetti, whole-wheat, dry (12 ounces)
- Sugar, confectioners' (1 ounce)
- Sugar, dark brown (1½ pounds)
- Sugar, light brown (11 ounces)
- Sugar, white (6 ounces)
- Sunflower seeds, unsalted (2½ ounces)
- Vermicelli, angel hair, or Mexican fideo noodles, whole-wheat, dry (4 ounces)
- Walnuts (2 ounces)
- Walnuts, cashews, or pistachios, unsalted raw or dry-roasted (1 ounce)

Refrigerated and Frozen Foods

- Corn kernels, frozen (5 ounces)
- Eggs, large (32)
- Lima beans, frozen (or fresh) (12 ounces)
- Sorbet, chocolate (4 ounces)
- Strawberries, frozen (10 ounces)

Other

- Bread, crusty, chewy whole-grain (1 small loaf)
- Bread, rye (1 small loaf)
- Chocolate, unsweetened baking (8 ounces)
- Chocolate, dark (1 ounce)
- Coffee, black (6 ounces)
- Graham crackers (8 pieces)
- Matzo, whole-wheat (1 piece)
- Tortillas, whole-wheat (5)

PLAN-AHEAD PREPARATIONS

This week there are several things you can prepare ahead of time and use throughout the week to make your life easier.

1. **Grains and Pasta.** Depending on the recipe, you may be able to cook your rice, quinoa, or pasta a day or more before using it. Especially when it comes to brown rice, which takes 45 to 50 minutes to cook, precooking can be a wonderful convenience. If you precook pasta, toss it in just a little olive oil before storing it to keep it from sticking. Give your grains a chance to cool completely before you put them in the fridge.

2. **Beans.** Many DASH recipes call for legumes such as black beans, chickpeas (garbanzo beans), white (navy) beans, and lima beans. You can buy canned, low-sodium varieties and drain and rinse them just before using, but you can save money and control your sodium better if you cook your own beans from scratch ahead of time. In the refrigerator, they'll keep for a day or two.

3. **Breakfasts.** You can make the filling for the Herbed Asparagus and Balsamic Onion Frittata a day in advance. Let it cool completely before putting it in the fridge in a sealed container.

4. **Lunches.** You can make any of the following a day or two in advance: Creamy Butternut-Apple Soup, Hearty Pasta Salad, and the protein portions of the Chicken-Grape Salad Sandwiches, Chicken-Lettuce Wraps with Spicy Soy Sauce, Fish Tacos, and Swanky Steak Sandwich. Allow the cooked ingredients to cool completely before you put them in the fridge in sealed containers or plastic zip-top bags.

5. **Side Dishes.** You can make any of the following a day in advance: Black Bean Confetti Salad, Perfect Coleslaw, Pilaf Parmesan, and Spanish-Style Sautéed Baby Spinach. The pilaf and spinach should be completely cool before you refrigerate them.

6. **Dinners.** You can make either of these a day in advance: Beef Stroganoff with Lemony Roasted Broccoli and Comforting Mac and Cheese with Lima Beans with Spinach. Cool them completely before putting them in sealed containers in the fridge.

7. **Dinner Elements.** You can make the compote for the Pork Scaloppini and the meat sauce for the spaghetti a day or two in advance.

8. **Desserts.** You can make any of the desserts a day or two in advance.

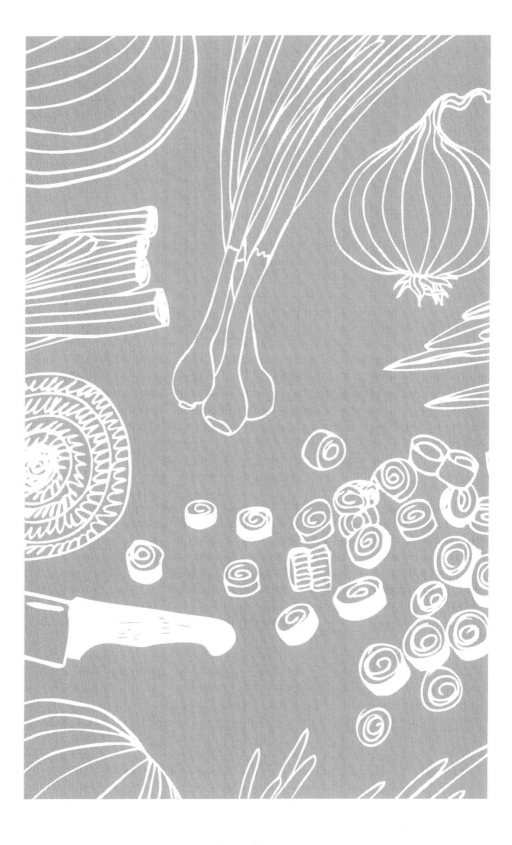

Week Three

Sodium not only affects your heart health, but your physical appearance as well. Excess sodium consumption may make your face feel puffy, give you bags under your eyes, increase swelling in your fingers, and make your jeans look, and feel, tighter. In fact, from an American Heart Association/ American Stroke Association consumer poll, 75 percent of respondents stated that their pants feeling too tight is their least favorite effect of bloating, which may be associated with excess sodium consumption.

—American Heart Association, "Salty Six: Common Foods Loaded with Excess Sodium"

WEEK THREE MEAL PLAN

Day One

Total sodium: 1,451 mg

Breakfast
Blueberry and Oat Pancakes
Sodium per serving: 288 mg
Lunch
Lentils and Kale over Brown Rice
Sodium per serving: 328 mg

Snack

½ cup shredded wheat with ½ cup 1 percent milk

Sodium per serving: 60 mg

Dinner

Turkey Meatloaf

Sodium per serving: 422 mg

Maple-Pecan Mashed Sweet Potatoes

Sodium per serving: 179 mg

Dessert

Frozen Chocolate–Peanut Butter Pudding Squares

Sodium per serving: 174 mg

. . . .

Daily Tip: Avocados are bursting with heart-healthful fat. Use them in place of bad fats in a wide range of dishes, from salads (think mayonnaise) to sandwiches (cheese) to baked goods (butter).

. . . .

Day Two

Total sodium: 1,354 mg

Breakfast

Tropical Strawberry Shake

Sodium per serving: 164 mg

Lunch

Chicken Quesadillas with Pico de Gallo

Sodium per serving: 309 mg

Snack

2 ounces unsalted whole-wheat pretzels

Sodium per serving: 180 mg

Dinner

Green Lasagna

Sodium per serving: 310 mg

Parmesan-Crusted Cauliflower

Sodium per serving: 209 mg

Dessert

Carrot-Raisin-Oatmeal Cookies

Sodium per serving: 182 mg

Daily Tip: Take control of the fiber, fat, and sodium in your bread crumbs by making your own. Dry slices of whole-grain bread in a 300°F oven for 10 to 15 minutes, then run them through a food processor or blender. You may season the crumbs and freeze them, all while reducing food waste and saving money.

Day Three

Total sodium: 1,242 mg

Breakfast
Red, White, and Blue Parfait
Sodium per serving: 62 mg
Lunch
Mini English Muffin Pizzas
Sodium per serving: 365 mg
Snack
3 cups unsalted air-popped popcorn sprinkled with chili powder
Sodium per serving: 2 mg
Dinner
Orange-Flavored Beef with Stir-Fried Vegetables
Sodium per serving: 390 mg
Brown Rice Pilaf
Sodium per serving: 178 mg
Dessert
Righteous Pumpkin Pie
Sodium per serving: 245 mg

Daily Tip: When you're shopping for meat, look for *loin* and *round* cuts of beef and pork, which are lower in fat. Check the USDA grade of beef: *choice* and *select* are less fatty, while *prime* cuts are fattier.

Day Four

Total sodium: 1,270 mg

Breakfast
Pecan and Sunflower Seed Granola
Sodium per serving: 150 mg
Lunch
Pepper Steak Salad
Sodium per serving: 584 mg
Snack
1 unsalted brown-rice cake with 2 ounces low-sodium cottage cheese
and 1 ounce blanched spinach
Sodium per serving: 152 mg
Dinner
Creamy Sole with Grapes
Sodium per serving: 193 mg
Aromatic Almond Couscous
Sodium per serving: 99 mg
Dessert
Chocolate–Sweet Potato Pudding
Sodium per serving: 92 mg

> **Daily Tip:** Extra-virgin olive oil might cost a little more than the other stuff, but it's full of cancer-fighting antioxidants because it's cold-pressed. Buy the best extra-virgin olive oil you can afford to get the biggest hit of antioxidants and flavor.

Day Five

Total sodium: 1,331 mg

Breakfast
Mediterranean Spinach Omelet
Sodium per serving: 441 mg

Lunch
Chicken-Lettuce Wraps with Spicy Soy Sauce
Sodium per serving: 297 mg
Snack
1 medium maple-cinnamon baked apple
Sodium per serving: 4 mg
Dinner
Three-Bean Chili
Sodium per serving: 469 mg
Zesty Quinoa
Sodium per serving: 103 mg
Dessert
Strawberry-Banana Frozen Yogurt
Sodium per serving: 17 mg

> **Daily Tip:** One cup of dried beans makes about three cups of cooked beans—about what you get from two drained 15-ounce cans.

Day Six

Total sodium: 1,391 mg

Breakfast
Apricot-Orange Bread
Sodium per serving: 228 mg
Lunch
Tuna-Apple Salad Sandwiches
Sodium per serving: 231 mg
Snack
½ cup halved cherry or grape tomatoes with 1 tablespoon crumbled reduced-fat feta cheese
Sodium per serving: 207 mg
Dinner
Baked BBQ Chicken
Sodium per serving: 497 mg
Jalapeño Cornbread
Sodium per serving: 103 mg

Dessert
The Original Flan
Sodium per serving: 125 mg

> **Daily Tip:** To make cutting vegetables, fruit, and proteins easier and safer, put a damp towel between your counter and your cutting board. That way, the board won't slip around while you work.

Day Seven

Total sodium: 1,359 mg

Breakfast
Peanut Butter and Banana Smoothie
Sodium per serving: 200 mg
Lunch
Southwestern Quinoa–Black Bean Salad
Sodium per serving: 315 mg
Snack
¼ cup unsalted raw or dry-roasted sunflower seeds or pumpkin seeds
Sodium per serving: 0 mg
Dinner
Chicken-Asparagus Penne
Sodium per serving: 476 mg
Tuscan Kale Salad Massaged with Roasted Garlic
Sodium per serving: 244 mg
Dessert
Heavenly Apple Crisp
Sodium per serving: 124 mg

> **Daily Tip:** Make your life simpler by making extra servings. Double a recipe, portion out the leftovers, and stash them in the freezer. Talk about convenience food!

ADDITIONAL TIPS FOR WEEK THREE

- The Nutrition Facts label on packaged foods is an excellent resource when you're following the DASH diet. Take note of the serving sizes used to measure the fat, carbohydrates, and other nutrients. If you're eating more than one serving, calculate your sodium, fat, and calorie intake accordingly.

- Confused about the different ways food labels describe sodium levels? Here's the fine print: Per serving, "low sodium" = less than 140 mg; "very low sodium" = less than 35 mg; and "sodium-free" = less than 5 mg. You may also see the terms "reduced sodium" or "less sodium," which means sodium has been reduced by at least 25 percent per serving, and "light," which means sodium has been reduced by at least 50 percent per serving.

- Boost the heart-healthful benefits you get from your salad. Dark green spinach, arugula, and watercress pack a bigger nutritional punch than lighter color greens such as romaine, iceberg, and Boston lettuce.

- Perhaps you're one of the many of people who react to stress by eating. When you're under pressure or your emotions are high, try diffusing the energy with action instead of food. Take a brisk walk, play with your pet, putter in your garden, or talk to a friend. Doing something you enjoy is likely to give you a lift and cancel your craving in as little as ten to fifteen minutes.

- Studies have shown that reducing sodium, refined sugar, and fat in your diet and adding whole grains, fresh produce, and lean proteins can increase the efficacy of your blood pressure and other medications. Eat right, and you might be able to cut back on or even throw out some of your medicine. Of course, talk to your doctor first.

WEEK THREE SHOPPING LIST

Pantry Items

- Baking powder
- Baking soda
- Basil, dried
- Black peppercorns
- Chili powder
- Cinnamon, ground
- Cocoa powder, unsweetened
- Coriander, ground
- Cornstarch
- Cumin, ground
- Ginger, ground
- Honey

- Maple syrup, pure
- Mustard, dry
- Nutmeg, ground
- Oil, canola
- Oil, extra-virgin olive
- Oil, sesame
- Oregano, dried
- Paprika
- Red pepper flakes, crushed (optional)
- Salt
- Tarragon, dried
- Vanilla extract, pure
- Vinegar, cider
- Vinegar, red wine

Produce

- Apples, medium (9)
- Arugula (1 pound)
- Asparagus (2 bunches, about 2 pounds)
- Bananas (5)
- Basil, fresh (1 bunch)
- Bell peppers, green (2)
- Bell peppers, red (3)
- Bell peppers, yellow (1)
- Blueberries (13 ounces)
- Broccoli head (2)
- Cabbage, Napa (Asian) or savoy (8 ounces)
- Carrots (6)
- Cauliflower, head (1)
- Celery (1 bunch)
- Cherries (8 ounces)
- Chives, fresh (1 bunch)
- Cilantro, fresh (1 bunch)
- Garlic (3 heads)
- Ginger, fresh (2 ounces)
- Grapes, seedless green (4 ounces)
- Jalapeño peppers (5)
- Kale, curly (2 bunches)
- Kale, Tuscan (4 bunches)
- Lemons (7)
- Lettuce head, Boston or butter (1)
- Lettuce, salad greens (8 ounces)
- Limes (4)
- Mushrooms, button or cremini (2 ounces)
- Mushrooms, shiitake (2 ounces)
- Onions, red (4)
- Onions, white or yellow (10)
- Oranges (2)
- Oregano, fresh (1 bunch)
- Parsley, fresh (1 bunch)
- Potatoes, sweet (4)
- Raspberries (8 ounces)
- Scallions (1 bunch)
- Spinach (6 ounces)
- Strawberries (5 ounces)
- Thyme, fresh (1 bunch)
- Tomatoes (4)
- Tomatoes, cherry (1 pound)
- Zucchini (1)

Protein

- Chicken breasts, boneless, skinless (nine, 3-ounce)
- Chicken drumsticks (two, 6-ounce)
- Chicken thighs, boneless, skinless (two, 3-ounce)
- Sole fillets (four, 3-ounce)
- Steak, flank (12 ounces)
- Steak, top round (1 pound)
- Tuna, low-sodium chunk light in water (two, 6-ounce cans)
- Turkey, lean ground (1 pound)

Dairy

- Buttermilk, 1 percent (8 ounces)
- Cheese, feta, reduced-fat, crumbled (1 ounce)
- Cheese, mozzarella, part-skim, shredded (5 ounces)
- Cheese, Parmesan, grated (3 ounces)
- Cheese, pepper Jack, shredded (2 ounces)
- Cottage cheese, low-sodium nonfat (1 pint)
- Margarine, soft tub (8 ounces)
- Milk, 1 percent (1 pint plus 8 ounces)
- Milk, skim (1 quart plus 1 pint)
- Yogurt, nonfat plain Greek (2 quarts)

Canned and Bottled Foods

- Applesauce, unsweetened (4 ounces)
- Beans, black, low-sodium (two, 15-ounce cans)
- Beans, pinto, low-sodium (15-ounce can)
- Beans, red kidney, low-sodium (15-ounce can)
- Broth, chicken, low-sodium (20 ounces)
- Evaporated milk, nonfat (6 ounces)
- Hoisin sauce (1½ ounces)
- Hot sauce (1 ounce)
- Ketchup, low-sodium (2½ ounces)
- Peanut butter, unsalted natural (2½ ounces)
- Pineapple, crushed in juice (two, 15-ounce cans)
- Pumpkin (15-ounce can)
- Soy sauce, low-sodium (2 ounces)
- Tomato paste, no salt added (6-ounce can)
- Tomato sauce, no salt added (three, 14.5-ounce cans)
- Tomatoes, diced, no salt added (28-ounce can)
- Worcestershire sauce (2 ounces)

Dry Foods

- Almonds, slivered (4 ounces)
- Apricots, dried (1 ounce)
- Bread crumbs, whole-wheat, no salt added (1 ounce)
- Coconut flakes, unsweetened (3 ounces)
- Cornmeal (7 ounces)
- Couscous, whole-wheat instant (7 ounces)
- Cranberries, dried unsweetened (2 ounces)
- Flour, unbleached all-purpose (12 ounces)
- Flour, whole-wheat (12 ounces)
- Graham cracker crumbs (1 ounce)
- Hazelnuts, unsalted (3 ounces)
- Instant espresso powder (1 teaspoon)
- Lasagna noodles, whole-wheat, dry (12 ounces)
- Lentils, brown, dry (7 ounces)
- Milk powder, nonfat (2 ounces)
- Oats, rolled (2½ pounds)
- Oats, steel-cut (3 ounces)
- Pecans (13 ounces)
- Penne, whole-wheat, dry (8 ounces)
- Popcorn, un-popped (1 ounce)
- Quinoa, dry (11 ounces)
- Raisins (7 ounces)
- Raisins, golden (4 ounces)
- Rice, brown, dry (1 pound)
- Sesame seeds (1 ounce)
- Sugar, light brown (11 ounces)
- Sugar, white (7 ounces)
- Sunflower seeds, unsalted raw or dry-roasted (4½ ounces)

Refrigerated and Frozen Foods

- Eggs (15)
- Strawberries, frozen (10 ounces)

Other

- Almond milk, unsweetened (4 ounces)
- Brown-rice cake, unsalted (1)
- English muffins, whole-wheat (4)
- Graham crackers (5-ounce package)
- Pita pockets, whole-wheat (2)
- Pretzels, whole-wheat, unsalted (2 ounces)
- Protein powder (1 ounce)
- Sherry, dry (optional) (½ ounce)
- Shredded wheat (4 ounces)
- Tortillas, whole-wheat (4)
- White wine, dry (4 ounces)

PLAN-AHEAD PREPARATIONS

This week there are several things you can prepare ahead of time and use throughout the week to make your life easier.

1. **Poultry and Meat.** When you can't the find poultry or meat butchered exactly as you need it, do the work yourself as soon as you get home from the store. Remove the skin from poultry and debone the breasts, and trim all visible fat from meat. Now is also a good time to portion out your protein for the week's recipes.

2. **Dressings and Marinades.** Most salad dressings and marinades can be prepared in advance. In fact, most of them taste better if they sit for a while before you use them.

3. **Lunches.** You can make any of the following a day or two in advance: Lentils and Kale over Brown Rice and Southwestern Quinoa–Black Bean Salad; the protein portions of the Chicken-Lettuce Wraps with Spicy Soy Sauce, Pepper Steak Salad, and Tuna-Apple Salad Sandwiches; and the pico de gallo for the Chicken Quesadillas. Allow hot items to cool completely before you put them in the fridge in sealed containers or plastic zip-top bags.

4. **Side Dishes.** You can make the Aromatic Almond Couscous and Brown Rice Pilaf a day in advance. Let them cool off and store them in the fridge in sealed containers or plastic zip-top bags.

5. **Entire Dinners.** You can make any of the following a day in advance: Baked BBQ Chicken with Jalapeño Cornbread, Green Lasagna with Parmesan-Crusted Cauliflower, Three-Bean Chili with Zesty Quinoa, and Turkey Meatloaf with Maple-Pecan Mashed Sweet Potatoes. Let everything cool completely before refrigerating it in sealed containers or plastic zip-top bags.

6. **Desserts.** You can make any of the desserts a day or two in advance.

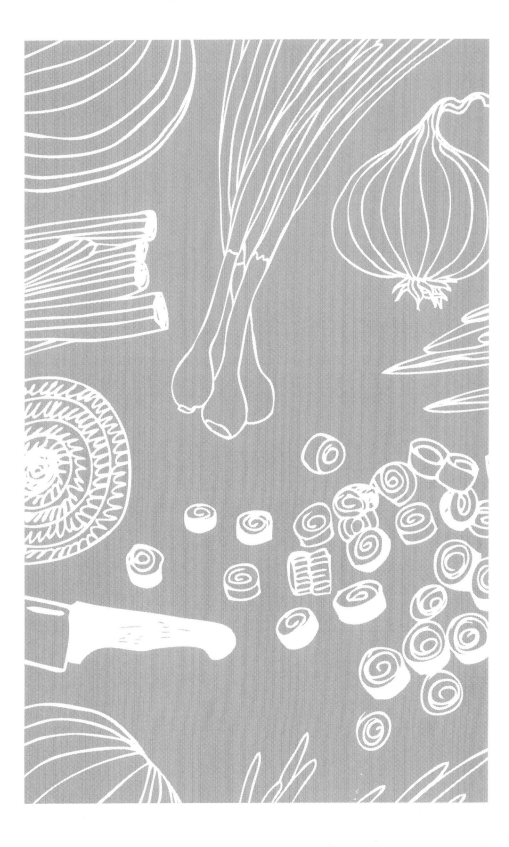

Week Four

The largest reductions in blood pressure [on the DASH diet] were found among three groups: people older than 45, patients with hypertension, and African-Americans. . . . The findings also hold significance for young people with normal blood pressure, because adopting these changes on a long-term basis may help blunt the increase in blood pressure that occurs with increasing age.

—John O'Neil, "A Diet That's Beneficial at Any Age"

WEEK FOUR MEAL PLAN

Day One

Total sodium: 1,510 mg

Breakfast
Honey-Walnut Fruit Salad
Sodium per serving: 3 mg
Lunch
Traditional Beef Stew
Sodium per serving: 607 mg
Snack
1 (12-ounce) vanilla-almond-oat protein shake
Sodium per serving: 65 mg

Dinner
Teriyaki Salmon Stir-Fry
Sodium per serving: 389 mg
Asian Noodles
Sodium per serving: 282 mg
Dessert
Death by Chocolate Cupcakes
Sodium per serving: 164 mg

. . . .

Daily Tip: When chopping vegetables, slicing fruit, or trimming meat, protect your fingers from cuts by curling the tips under and holding the food against the cutting board with your first knuckles. Instead of bringing the knife toward you as you chop, push the food toward the knife.

. . . .

Day Two

Total sodium: 1,549 mg

Breakfast
Apple-Cinnamon Oatmeal
Sodium per serving: 293 mg
Lunch
Bulgur and Chickpea Salad
Sodium per serving: 256 mg
Snack
¼ cup salsa with 1 ounce unsalted tortilla chips
Sodium per serving: 50 mg
Dinner
Beef Stroganoff
Sodium per serving: 538 mg
Lemony Roasted Broccoli
Sodium per serving: 320 mg
Dessert
Chocolate–Sweet Potato Pudding
Sodium per serving: 92 mg

Day Three

Total sodium: 1,385 mg

Breakfast
Pecan and Sunflower Seed Granola
Sodium per serving: 150 mg
Lunch
Turkey Noodle Soup
Sodium per serving: 434 mg
Snack
1 tablespoon unsalted natural almond butter on 1 slice whole-grain bread
Sodium per serving: 130 mg
Dinner
Pork Scaloppini with Apple-Raisin Compote
Sodium per serving: 200 mg
Pilaf Parmesan
Sodium per serving: 317 mg
Dessert
Fudgy Cookies
Sodium per serving: 154 mg

Day Four

Total sodium: 1,411 mg

Breakfast
Blueberry and Oat Pancakes
Sodium per serving: 288 mg
Lunch
Swanky Steak Sandwich
Sodium per serving: 391 mg
Snack
¾ cup cantaloupe and grape salad with lemon and mint
Sodium per serving: 4 mg
Dinner
Comforting Mac and Cheese
Sodium per serving: 192 mg
Lima Beans with Spinach
Sodium per serving: 362 mg
Dessert
Frozen Chocolate–Peanut Butter Pudding Squares
Sodium per serving: 174 mg

. . . .

Daily Tip: Chocoholics, rejoice! Dark chocolate, with its high cacao content, is packed with a type of nutrient called flavonoids, which can protect you from heart disease.

. . . .

Day Five

Total sodium: 1,465 mg

Breakfast
Tropical Strawberry Shake
Sodium per serving: 164 mg
Lunch
Hearty Pasta Salad
Sodium per serving: 370 mg

Snack

2 pieces (1 ounce each) tuna, salmon, or yellowtail sashimi with a dash of soy sauce and ¼ teaspoon prepared wasabi

Sodium per serving: 115 mg

Dinner

Crispy Thanksgiving Turkey Fillets

Sodium per serving: 510 mg

Cinnamon-Roasted Glazed Carrots

Sodium per serving: 124 mg

Dessert

Carrot-Raisin-Oatmeal Cookies

Sodium per serving: 182 mg

Daily Tip: If you're a pasta fan, you might need a little time to adjust to the whole-wheat varieties. They're a bit chewier and have a slightly rougher texture than white pasta, but they also have a wonderful nutty quality. You can ease your transition by trying a whole-white hybrid pasta first.

Day Six

Total sodium: 1,538 mg

Breakfast

Red, White, and Blue Parfait

Sodium per serving: 62 mg

Lunch

Fish Tacos

Sodium per serving: 395 mg

Snack

1 cup cooked oatmeal with 1 tablespoon dried cranberries

Sodium per serving: 297 mg

Dinner

Spaghetti with Meat Sauce

Sodium per serving: 440 mg

Spanish-Style Sautéed Baby Spinach

Sodium per serving: 180 mg

Dessert
Death by Chocolate Cupcakes
Sodium per serving: 164 mg

. . . .

Daily Tip: When cooking or baking with eggs, you can get all the binding and leavening characteristics of whole eggs by using egg whites, which are available in small cartons at the supermarket, usually right near the eggs. Do some experimenting; in many cases, two egg whites can take the place of one whole egg.

. . . .

Day Seven

Total sodium: 1,593 mg

Breakfast
Herbed Asparagus and Balsamic Onion Frittata
Sodium per serving: 396 mg

Lunch
Chicken-Grape Salad Sandwiches
Sodium per serving: 350 mg

Snack
1 piece (1 ounce) low-sodium string cheese
Sodium per serving: 200 mg

Dinner
Beef Tenderloin Mole
Sodium per serving: 226 mg

Black Bean Confetti Salad
Sodium per serving: 176 mg

Dessert
Righteous Pumpkin Pie
Sodium per serving: 245 mg

. . . .

Daily Tip: Got the munchies? You might be surprised to discover how little it takes to satisfy your sweet tooth. Cut up bite-size pieces of your favorite candies, cookies, cakes, and even ice cream, seal the pieces in plastic wrap, and freeze them. When the sugarplum fairy comes knocking, pop a morsel into your mouth and let the sweetness melt over your tongue. Voilà!

ADDITIONAL TIPS FOR WEEK FOUR

- Eating well is about quality, not quantity. You will enjoy your food more and find your meals more satisfying if you focus on the flavors on your plate and share them with family and friends. Slow down and savor!
- Broaden your culinary horizons and add more texture and color to your meals by trying nonmeat proteins such as legumes and tofu. These ingredients soak up the flavors of sauces, spices, and herbs, with delicious results. One cup of cooked legumes or tofu does the job, protein-wise, of two ounces of fish, poultry, or meat.
- Many diet plans advise you to eat five small meals a day instead of three large ones. The DASH diet is designed to keep your metabolism fueled throughout the day but doesn't dictate how many meals you should have. As long as you don't overeat and you spread your meals over the course of the day, you can split your intake into as many meals as works best for you.
- Eat fish at least twice a week. The omega-3 fatty acids in creatures that swim are good for your cardiovascular system. And like your mother always told you, fish is brain food.
- Changing your habits is hard, and switching over to the DASH diet will have its challenges. Like everyone else, you'll have your lapses. But just because you stumble doesn't mean you'll fall. When you do slip, forgive and forget, and get back on track.

WEEK FOUR SHOPPING LIST

Pantry Items

- Arrowroot powder
- Baking powder
- Baking soda

- Basil, dried
- Black peppercorns
- Chili powder

- Cinnamon, ground
- Cocoa powder, unsweetened
- Coriander, ground
- Cornstarch
- Cumin, ground
- Ginger, ground
- Honey
- Maple syrup, pure
- Marjoram, dried
- Mirin
- Mustard, dry
- Nutmeg, ground
- Oil, canola
- Oil, extra-virgin olive
- Oil, sesame
- Oregano, dried
- Red pepper flakes, crushed
- Rosemary, dried
- Sage, dried
- Salt
- Tarragon, dried
- Thyme, dried
- Vanilla extract, pure
- Vinegar, balsamic
- Vinegar, cider
- Vinegar, rice

Produce

- Apples, medium (3)
- Asparagus (1 bunch, about 1 pound)
- Bananas (3)
- Basil, fresh (1 bunch)
- Bell peppers, red (3)
- Bell peppers, yellow (2)
- Blueberries (1½ pounds)
- Broccoli heads (2)
- Cabbage, green (4 ounces)
- Cantaloupe (1)
- Carrots (20)
- Celery (1 bunch)
- Cherries (8 ounces)
- Cilantro, fresh (1 bunch)
- Cucumber (1)
- Fennel bulb (1)
- Garlic (3 heads)
- Ginger, fresh (4 ounces)
- Grapes, seedless green (1 pound)
- Jalapeño peppers (3)
- Lemons (7)
- Lettuce head, romaine (1)
- Lettuce, salad greens (4 ounces)
- Limes (7)
- Mango (1)
- Mint, fresh (1 bunch)
- Mung bean sprouts (4 ounces)
- Mushrooms, button or cremini (11 ounces)
- Nectarine (1)
- Onions, red (3)
- Onions, white or yellow (8)
- Parsley, fresh (1 bunch)
- Peas, snap or snow (6 ounces)
- Potato, white (1)
- Potatoes, sweet (2)
- Raspberries (8 ounces)
- Sage, fresh (1 bunch)
- Scallions (2 bunches)
- Spinach (2 pounds)
- Squash, yellow (1)

- Strawberries (1 pound)
- Tarragon, fresh (1 bunch)
- Thyme, fresh (1 bunch)
- Tomato (1)
- Tomatoes, cherry (1 pound)
- Zucchini (1)

Protein

- Beef, ground, extra-lean (1 pound)
- Beef, tenderloin roast (1 pound)
- Beef, top round (1 pound)
- Chicken breasts, boneless, skinless (1½ pounds)
- Pork tenderloin (2-pound package)
- Salmon fillets (eight, 3-ounce)
- Sashimi; tuna, salmon, or yellow-tail (two, 1-ounce pieces)
- Steak, top round (12 ounces)
- Steak, top sirloin (8 ounces)
- Turkey breast fillets, skinless (four, 3-ounce)
- Turkey, small whole (1)

Dairy

- Buttermilk, 1 percent (8 ounces)
- Cheese, sharp cheddar, low-fat, finely shredded (6 ounces)
- Cheese, Parmesan, grated (3 ounces)
- Cheese, string, low-sodium (1-ounce piece)
- Margarine, soft tub (5 ounces)
- Milk, 1 percent (12 ounces)
- Milk, skim (1 quart)
- Yogurt, nonfat plain Greek (1 quart plus 8 ounces)

Canned and Bottled Foods

- Almond butter, unsalted natural (½ ounce)
- Applesauce, unsweetened (4 ounces)
- Beans, black, low-sodium (15-ounce can)
- Broth, beef, low-sodium (8 ounces)
- Broth, chicken, low-sodium (12 ounces)
- Chickpeas, low-sodium (two, 15-ounce cans)
- Dijon mustard (½ ounce)
- Evaporated milk, nonfat (10 ounces)
- Mayonnaise, light (3 ounces)
- Peanut butter, unsalted natural (2 ounces)
- Pineapple, crushed in juice (15-ounce can)
- Pineapple, diced in juice (15-ounce can)
- Pumpkin (15-ounce can)

- Soy sauce, low-sodium
  (1½ ounces)
- Tomatoes, crushed, no salt added
  (28-ounce can)
- Tomatoes, diced, no salt added
  (14.5-ounce can)
- Worcestershire sauce (½ ounce)

Dry Foods

- Asian brown rice vermicelli,
  dry (8 ounces)
- Bread crumbs, whole-wheat,
  no salt added (1 ounce)
- Bulgur, coarse, dry (7 ounces)
- Buttermilk powder (2 ounces)
- Coconut flakes, unsweetened
  (3 ounces)
- Cranberries, dried unsweetened
  (1 ounce)
- Egg noodles, whole-wheat, dry
  (12 ounces)
- Flour, unbleached all-purpose
  (8 ounces)
- Flour, whole-wheat (11 ounces)
- Flour, whole-wheat pastry
  (9 ounces)
- Graham cracker crumbs (1 ounce)
- Instant espresso powder
  (1 teaspoon)
- Macaroni, whole-wheat, dry
  (4 ounces)
- Milk powder, nonfat (2 ounces)
- Oatmeal, cooked (8 ounces)
- Oats, rolled (2 pounds)
- Oats, steel-cut (11 ounces)
- Pasta shapes, tiny whole-wheat,
  dry (8 ounces)
- Pasta shapes, whole-wheat
  (8 ounces)
- Pecans (8 ounces)
- Pine nuts (pignoli), toasted
  (2 ounces)
- Raisins (10 ounces)
- Raisins, golden (3 ounces)
- Rice, white, long-grain, dry
  (7 ounces)
- Spaghetti, whole-wheat, dry
  (12 ounces)
- Sugar, confectioners' (1 ounce)
- Sugar, dark brown (1 pound)
- Sugar, light brown (13 ounces)
- Sugar, white (6 ounces)
- Sunflower seeds, unsalted
  (2½ ounces)
- Vermicelli, angel hair, or Mexican
  fideo noodles, whole-wheat, dry
  (4 ounces)
- Walnuts (2 ounces)

Refrigerated and Frozen Foods

- Corn kernels, frozen (5 ounces)
- Eggs (23)
- Lima beans, frozen (or fresh)
  (12 ounces)

Other

- Almond milk, unsweetened (16 ounces)
- Bread, crusty, chewy, whole-grain (1 small loaf)
- Bread, rye (1 small loaf)
- Chocolate, baking, unsweetened (4 ounces)
- Coffee, black (12 ounces)
- Cornbread (see Chapter 9) (4-by-4-inch square)
- Graham crackers (5-ounce package)
- Protein powder (1 ounce)
- Tortilla chips, unsalted (1 ounce)
- Tortillas, whole-wheat (4)
- Wasabi, prepared (¼ teaspoon)

PLAN-AHEAD PREPARATIONS

This week there are several things you can prepare ahead of time and use throughout the week to make your life easier.

1. **Fresh Lemon Juice.** Lemon juice is a superb replacement for salt. Keep some on hand for the many times that you will need it throughout the week. Get out that juicer and squeeze several lemons at a time.

2. **Fruit.** You can't have too much prepared fruit on hand, especially at breakfast. It's no fun to do a lot of kitchen work first thing in the morning, so get a batch of fruit ready every few days. Core and slice strawberries, pick grapes off of their bunches, de-stem and pit cherries, and peel and segment oranges. If you cut up apples more than half an hour before using them, toss them in a plastic zip-top bag so they don't go brown.

3. **Overripe Bananas.** When a recipe calls for very ripe bananas, and there aren't any in your produce section, buy what's available a few days ahead of time and let them sit on the counter until their peels begin to darken with spots.

4. **Lunches.** You can make any of the following a day or two in advance: Bulgur and Chickpea Salad, Hearty Pasta Salad, Traditional Beef Stew, and Turkey Noodle Soup; and the protein portions of the Chicken-Grape Salad Sandwiches, Fish Tacos, and Swanky Steak Sandwich. Allow the hot ingredients to cool completely before storing them in the fridge in sealed containers or plastic zip-top bags.

5. **Side Dishes.** You can make any of the following a day in advance: Cinnamon-Roasted Glazed Carrots, Pilaf Parmesan, and Spanish-Style Sautéed Baby Spinach. Give them a chance to cool completely; then put them in the fridge in plastic zip-top bags or sealed containers.

6. **Entire Dinners.** You can make either of the following a day in advance: Beef Stroganoff with Lemony Roasted Broccoli and Comforting Mac and Cheese with Lima Beans with Spinach. Cool the dishes completely and seal them in airtight containers or plastic zip-top bags; then refrigerate them.

7. **Dinner Elements.** You can make the compote for the Pork Scaloppini and the meat sauce for the spaghetti a day or two in advance. Keep them in the fridge after they've cooled completely.

8. **Dessert.** You can make any of the desserts a day or two in advance.

PART THREE

DASH Diet Recipes

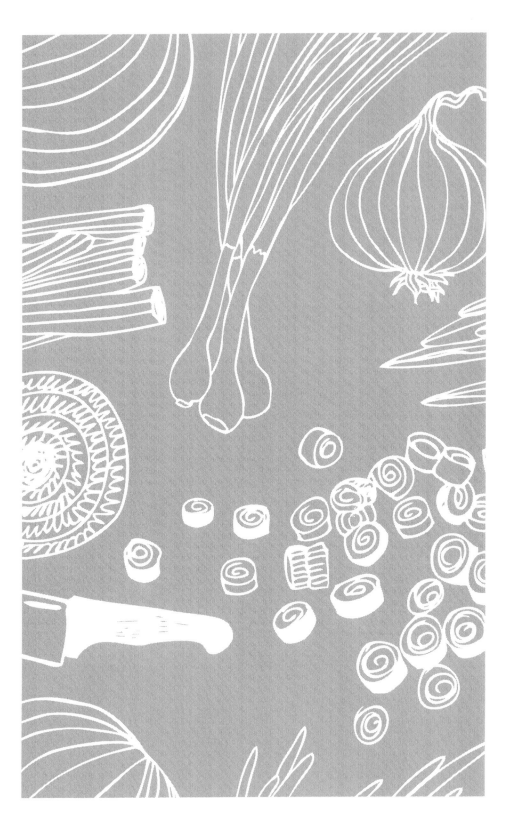

CHAPTER SEVEN

DASH Breakfasts

TROPICAL STRAWBERRY SHAKE

PEANUT BUTTER AND BANANA SMOOTHIE

HONEY-WALNUT FRUIT SALAD

RED, WHITE, AND BLUE PARFAIT

APPLE-CINNAMON OATMEAL

PECAN AND SUNFLOWER SEED GRANOLA

HERBED ASPARAGUS AND BALSAMIC ONION FRITTATA

MEDITERRANEAN SPINACH OMELET

BLUEBERRY AND OAT PANCAKES

APRICOT-ORANGE BREAD

Tropical Strawberry Shake

Calories per serving: 221

▸   SODIUM PER SERVING: 164 MG

Some mornings, you can't seem to shake off that sleepiness. You don't have to reach for the coffee; this refreshing, chilled fruit shake will wake you up. The protein will keep you going all morning, too.

1 CUP NONFAT PLAIN GREEK YOGURT

6 STRAWBERRIES

1 CUP CRUSHED PINEAPPLE, CANNED IN JUICE

1 RIPE BANANA, PEELED AND SLICED

1 TEASPOON PURE VANILLA EXTRACT

1 SCOOP PROTEIN POWDER (YOUR CHOICE)

6 ICE CUBES

1. Put all the ingredients in a blender and process until smooth.

2. Serve the shake immediately in tall glasses with straws.

Peanut Butter and Banana Smoothie

SERVES 1 (SERVING SIZE IS 1¼ CUPS)

Calories per serving: 260

▸ SODIUM PER SERVING: 200 MG

Rich and silky, this smoothie really tames morning hunger pangs. To make it almost sinful, add a little unsweetened cocoa powder. Elvis (a big fan of peanut butter and banana sandwiches) would have loved this!

1 CUP SKIM MILK
½ CUP PEELED, SLICED BANANA
1 TABLESPOON UNSALTED NATURAL PEANUT BUTTER
½ TEASPOON PURE VANILLA EXTRACT
1 TEASPOON UNSWEETENED COCOA POWDER (OPTIONAL)
4 ICE CUBES

1. Put all the ingredients in a blender and process until smooth.

2. Serve the smoothie immediately in a tall glass with a straw.

Honey-Walnut Fruit Salad

SERVES 4 (SERVING SIZE IS 1¼ CUPS)

Calories per serving: 172

▶ SODIUM PER SERVING: 3 MG

The many colors and textures of the fruit in this salad make it a festive start to your day. Topped with walnuts for some crunch and protein, the salad gets a little extra fun from a drizzle of honey. For variety, try it with different fruits.

½ CUP CUBED MANGO

1 CUP BLUEBERRIES

1 BANANA, PEELED AND SLICED

1 CUP HALVED STRAWBERRIES

1 CUP SEEDLESS GREEN GRAPES

1 NECTARINE, PITTED AND CUT INTO THIN WEDGES

4 TABLESPOONS COARSELY CHOPPED WALNUTS

4 TEASPOONS HONEY

1. In a large mixing bowl, toss the fruit together.

2. Spoon the salad into 4 serving bowls and top each with 1 tablespoon of walnuts.

3. Drizzle each serving with 1 teaspoon of honey, and serve.

Red, White, and Blue Parfait

SERVES 4

Calories per serving: 164

► SODIUM PER SERVING: 62 MG

Get into the Fourth of July spirit with this breakfast dish. Perfect for summer, it takes advantage of the season's freshest fruit, but you may enjoy it any time of year with thawed frozen berries. The multicolored layers of the parfait will have you celebrating the Stars and Stripes.

1 CUP PITTED AND HALVED CHERRIES
2 CUPS NONFAT PLAIN GREEK YOGURT
1 CUP BLUEBERRIES
1 CUP RASPBERRIES
4 TEASPOONS HONEY

1. In each of 4 glasses, layer ¼ cup of cherries, 3 tablespoons of yogurt, ¼ cup of blueberries, 3 tablespoons of yogurt, ¼ cup of raspberries, and 2 tablespoons of yogurt.

2. Drizzle each parfait with 1 teaspoon of honey, and serve.

Apple-Cinnamon Oatmeal

SERVES 2 (SERVING SIZE IS 1½ CUPS)

Calories per serving: 284

▶ SODIUM PER SERVING: 293 MG

Oats are wildly good for you, with proven health benefits that range from lowering your cholesterol and reducing your risk of cardiovascular disease and heart failure to strengthening your immune system and protecting you from diabetes and certain cancers. Oatmeal is a perfect weight-loss food, too, stabilizing your blood sugar and filling you up with healthful fiber. Plus, it's just plain yummy.

¾ CUP STEEL-CUT OATS
2¼ CUPS WATER
¼ TEASPOON SALT
2 TABLESPOONS RAISINS
1 APPLE, PEELED, CORED, AND CHOPPED
1 TEASPOON GROUND CINNAMON

1. In a medium saucepan over medium heat, combine the oats, water, and salt. Bring the mixture to a boil; then reduce the heat to low. Simmer for 10 minutes, stirring often.

2. Mix in the raisins, apple, and cinnamon and cook for 5 to 10 more minutes, stirring often, until the oatmeal reaches the consistency you like.

3. Serve the oatmeal in cereal bowls.

Pecan and Sunflower Seed Granola

SERVES 12 (SERVING SIZE IS ½ CUP)

Calories per serving: 274

▸ SODIUM PER SERVING: 150 MG

Homemade granola beats store-bought hands down in terms of flavor, texture, and nutrition. Your kitchen will smell fantastic while this is baking. No matter the time of day, you might just have to make granola your next meal.

3 CUPS ROLLED OATS

1 CUP CHOPPED PECANS

½ CUP UNSALTED SUNFLOWER SEEDS

½ CUP UNSWEETENED COCONUT FLAKES

1½ TEASPOONS GROUND CINNAMON

¼ CUP HONEY

¼ CUP MELTED TUB MARGARINE

½ TEASPOON SALT

⅔ CUP RAISINS

1. Preheat the oven to 350°F.

2. In a large mixing bowl, thoroughly combine all the ingredients except the raisins.

3. Spread the mixture evenly on a large baking sheet and bake for 25 to 30 minutes, stirring every 5 minutes, until the granola is golden brown.

4. Remove the pan from the oven and mix in the raisins.

5. Allow the granola to cool completely before storing it in an airtight container.

6. Serve the granola in cereal bowls, with skim milk or nonfat Greek yogurt.

Herbed Asparagus and Balsamic Onion Frittata

SERVES 4

Calories per serving: 149

▶ SODIUM PER SERVING: 396 MG

Packed with protein and vegetables, this is a great low-carb dish. Serve it with fruit salad on the side for a beautiful Sunday brunch. Or you may make the frittata whenever you have the time and refrigerate it in an airtight container until you're ready to reheat and eat.

1 TABLESPOON EXTRA-VIRGIN OLIVE OIL

1 WHITE OR YELLOW ONION, THINLY SLICED

2 TEASPOONS BALSAMIC VINEGAR

1 BUNCH (ABOUT 1 POUND) ASPARAGUS, WOODY ENDS CUT OFF AND
    GREEN STALKS CUT DIAGONALLY INTO 1-INCH PIECES

½ TEASPOON SALT, DIVIDED

2 TABLESPOONS WATER

4 EGGS

3 EGG WHITES

2 TABLESPOONS CHOPPED FRESH TARRAGON

2 TABLESPOONS CHOPPED FRESH PARSLEY

FRESHLY GROUND BLACK PEPPER

1. Preheat the broiler to high.

2. In a large, ovenproof skillet over medium heat, heat the oil. Add the onions and sauté until they are softened and golden brown, about 5 minutes.

3. Add the vinegar, asparagus, ¼ teaspoon of salt, and water, cover the pan, and steam until the vegetables are crisp-tender, about 3 minutes.

4. Remove the cover from the skillet and continue cooking until the liquid is almost gone.

5. While the vegetables cook, whisk together the eggs, egg whites, herbs, and remaining ¼ teaspoon of salt in a medium bowl and season it with the pepper.

6. Pour the egg mixture into the skillet with the asparagus and onions and stir to combine. Cook for 2 minutes.

7. Transfer the skillet to the broiler and cook until the frittata is lightly browned, about 3 minutes.

8. Remove the pan from the broiler and let the frittata rest for 3 minutes.

9. Slide the frittata onto a cutting board, cut it into 4 equal portions, and serve.

Mediterranean Spinach Omelet

SERVES 1

Calories per serving: 150

▸ SODIUM PER SERVING: 441 MG

Close your eyes, and the flavors of feta and oregano will transport you to the Greek Isles. This isn't a low-sodium dish, but if that worries you, you may leave out the feta. If not, and you're in more of an Italian mood, switch out the feta for freshly grated Parmesan cheese.

1 EGG
2 EGG WHITES
1 TEASPOON EXTRA-VIRGIN OLIVE OIL
½ CUP SLICED BUTTON OR CREMINI MUSHROOMS
1 CUP CHOPPED SPINACH
2 TABLESPOONS CRUMBLED FETA CHEESE
1 TEASPOON CHOPPED FRESH OREGANO
FRESHLY GROUND BLACK PEPPER

1. In a small bowl, whisk the egg with the egg whites. Set aside.

2. In a medium skillet over medium heat, heat the olive oil. Add the mushrooms and sauté until they give up their liquid, about 4 minutes.

3. Add the spinach and cook until it wilts, 2 to 3 minutes. Transfer the mixture to a small bowl, cover to keep it warm, and set aside.

4. Pour the egg mixture into the skillet and cook until the outer edges set. Use a spatula to loosen the edges from the pan. Lift the edges at several points around the pan and tilt the pan so the uncooked egg runs under the cooked egg.

5. When the eggs are mostly set, scatter the feta and sautéed spinach and mushrooms over the top. Sprinkle on the oregano and season with pepper.

6. Fold the omelet in half and cook for 1 minute.

7. Serve immediately.

Blueberry and Oat Pancakes

SERVES 4 (SERVING SIZE IS ABOUT 3 LARGE PANCAKES)

Calories per serving: 440

▶ SODIUM PER SERVING: 288 MG

Just because you're trimming down and shaping up doesn't mean you have to forego your morning pancakes. High in fiber and big on protein, these are perfect breakfast fuel that will get you to lunch before you know it. If you want to knock down the sodium, substitute applesauce for the yogurt.

½ CUP STEEL-CUT OATS
1½ CUPS WATER
1 CUP WHOLE-WHEAT FLOUR
½ TEASPOON BAKING POWDER
½ TEASPOON BAKING SODA
1 EGG
1 CUP 1 PERCENT MILK
½ CUP NONFAT PLAIN GREEK YOGURT
1 TEASPOON PURE VANILLA EXTRACT
1 CUP BLUEBERRIES (FRESH OR THAWED FROZEN)
2 TEASPOONS CANOLA OIL
½ CUP PURE MAPLE SYRUP

1. In a medium saucepan over medium heat, combine the oats and water. Bring the mixture to a boil; then reduce the heat to low. Simmer for 15 minutes, stirring often. Remove the pot from the heat and set aside.

2. In a medium bowl, combine the flour, baking powder, baking soda, egg, milk, yogurt, and vanilla extract. Mix until just smooth; do not overmix.

3. Stir the oatmeal to loosen it up; then mix it into the batter along with the blueberries.

continued ▶

4. On a griddle or in a skillet over medium heat, heat ½ teaspoon of the canola oil. Working in batches, use a measuring cup to pour about ¼ cup of batter per pancake onto the griddle. Cook until the batter bubbles on top and the pancakes are golden on the bottom, 2 to 3 minutes. Flip the pancakes and cook for another 2 minutes. Transfer the pancakes to a warm plate and cover them with foil or a clean kitchen towel to keep them warm.

5. Repeat until all the batter is used up.

6. Divide the batch of pancakes into 4 equal portions and serve them with maple syrup on the side.

7. Refrigerate any leftover pancakes in an airtight container until you are ready to reheat and eat.

Apricot-Orange Bread

SERVES 9 (SERVING SIZE IS ONE 1-INCH SLICE)

Calories per serving: 222

▸ SODIUM PER SERVING: 228 MG

Each serving of this bread is a little slice of sunshine. Filled with tender apricots and crunchy pecans, it's a delightful opener to any day. Even though white flour is on the list of foods to avoid, it's used in moderation here for texture; there's some white sugar as well.

¼ CUP CHOPPED DRIED APRICOTS

1 CUP WATER

1 CUP UNBLEACHED ALL-PURPOSE FLOUR

¾ CUP WHOLE-WHEAT FLOUR

¼ CUP NONFAT DRY MILK POWDER

1 TEASPOON BAKING POWDER

½ TEASPOON BAKING SODA

½ TEASPOON SALT

1 TABLESPOON TUB MARGARINE

½ CUP SUGAR

1 EGG, LIGHTLY BEATEN

1½ TEASPOONS ORANGE ZEST

¼ CUP ORANGE JUICE

½ CUP CHOPPED PECANS

½ TEASPOON CANOLA OIL

1. Preheat the oven to 350°F.

2. In a medium saucepan over medium heat, combine the apricots and the water. Cover the pot and simmer until the apricots are plump and soften slightly, 10 to 15 minutes.

3. Drain the apricots, reserving ⅓ cup of liquid. Set aside.

continued ▸

4. Into a medium bowl, sift together the flours, milk powder, baking powder, baking soda, and salt.

5. In a large bowl, combine the margarine and sugar. Using a spoon, beat in the egg, orange zest, and orange juice.

6. In three batches, add the flour mixture and then the reserved apricot liquid to the margarine mixture until just combined. Mix the apricots and pecans into the batter.

7. Use the oil to grease the sides and bottom of a 9-by-5-inch loaf pan. Pour the batter into the pan.

8. Bake the loaf for 40 to 45 minutes, until the center of the loaf springs back when gently touched in the center.

9. Place the pan on a wire rack and allow the bread to cool for 5 minutes.

10. Slide a knife around the edges of the loaf before inverting the pan onto the rack to release the bread. Cool the bread completely before cutting it into 9 slices.

11. Wrap the bread in foil and refrigerate or freeze it until ready to eat.

CHAPTER EIGHT

DASH Lunches

Pepper Steak Salad

SERVES 4 (SERVING SIZE IS ABOUT 2 CUPS)

Calories per serving: 261

▸ SODIUM PER SERVING: 584 MG

Refreshing and satisfying at the same time, this salad is a must for steak lovers. The combination of protein and fiber will keep you feeling full all afternoon. If you're not going to serve a portion of it immediately, prevent the arugula from wilting by refrigerating the dressing, steak, and salad in three separate containers. Combine the ingredients when you're ready to eat.

FOR THE DRESSING:

¼ CUP CIDER VINEGAR

1 TEASPOON HONEY

½ TEASPOON HOT SAUCE

¼ TEASPOON FRESHLY GROUND BLACK PEPPER

2 TABLESPOONS EXTRA-VIRGIN OLIVE OIL

¼ CUP CHOPPED FRESH CHIVES

FOR THE SALAD:

1 RED ONION, CUT INTO ½-INCH SLICES

1 RED BELL PEPPER, SEEDED AND CUT INTO QUARTERS

1 YELLOW BELL PEPPER, SEEDED AND CUT INTO QUARTERS

2 TEASPOONS EXTRA-VIRGIN OLIVE OIL

1 POUND TOP ROUND STEAK, VISIBLE FAT TRIMMED

½ TEASPOON FRESHLY GROUND BLACK PEPPER

¼ TEASPOON SALT

4 CUPS CHOPPED ARUGULA

1 CUP HALVED CHERRY TOMATOES

To make the dressing:

In a medium bowl, whisk all the ingredients together until they are completely mixed. Set aside.

To make the salad:

1. Preheat the broiler or grill to medium-high (375°F to 450°F).

2. In separate medium bowls, toss the onion and bell peppers with 1 teaspoon of oil each.

3. Broil or grill the onions on one side for 5 minutes.

4. Turn the onions over and add the bell peppers, flesh side up, to the broiler pan or grill grate. Cook the vegetables for 5 minutes; then turn them over and continue cooking until they are tender and lightly charred, about 5 more minutes.

5. Transfer the vegetables to a cutting board and allow them to cool enough to handle. Cut the onions into quarters and separate the rings into crescents. Cut the peppers into 1/2-inch-wide strips. Set aside.

6. Sprinkle the steak all over with black pepper and salt. Broil or grill the meat until it reaches the desired temperature (about 4 minutes per side for medium-rare).

7. Transfer the steak to a cutting board and let it rest for 5 minutes.

8. Cut the steak against the grain into 1/4-inch-thick slices. Cut each slice in half, crosswise. Put the meat and its juice in a medium bowl.

9. Whisk the salad dressing again for a few seconds and add 2 tablespoons of the dressing to the bowl with the steak. Toss to coat the meat.

10. In a large bowl, toss the cooked vegetables with the arugula, tomatoes, and the rest of the dressing until everything is coated.

11. Divide the salad into equal portions on 4 serving plates. Top each with one-quarter of the steak, and serve.

Hearty Pasta Salad

SERVES 4 (SERVING SIZE IS ABOUT 1¾ CUPS)

Calories per serving: 390

▶ SODIUM PER SERVING: 370 MG

When lunchtime finds you extra-hungry, this salad is sure to fill you up. It's tastiest if you don't cook the pasta until it's soft because soft pasta will get mushy when it's combined with the other salad ingredients. Instead, cook it al dente, an Italian term that means "to the tooth"—still somewhat firm in the center.

8 OUNCES WHOLE-WHEAT PASTA SHAPES, SUCH AS FARFALLE
    (BOW TIES), ROTELLE (WAGON WHEELS), OR ROTINI (SPIRALS)

2 CUPS HALVED CHERRY TOMATOES

1 CUP SEEDED, ROUGHLY CHOPPED YELLOW BELL PEPPER

1 CUP SHREDDED ZUCCHINI

1 (15-OUNCE) CAN LOW-SODIUM CHICKPEAS, DRAINED, RINSED, AND
    SHAKEN DRY

1 TABLESPOON EXTRA-VIRGIN OLIVE OIL

2 TABLESPOONS BALSAMIC VINEGAR

1 TABLESPOON JULIENNED FRESH BASIL

¼ TEASPOON SALT

⅛ TEASPOON FRESHLY GROUND BLACK PEPPER

½ CUP GRATED PARMESAN CHEESE, DIVIDED

1. Cook the pasta al dente, according to the directions on the package, with no salt added. Drain and rinse the pasta in a colander under cold running water until the pasta is cool.

2. In a large bowl, toss together the vegetables, chickpeas, oil, vinegar, basil, salt, and pepper.

3. Add the pasta and toss gently to coat.

4. Divide the salad into equal portions on 4 serving plates. Top each with 2 tablespoons of cheese.

5. To save the salad for later, mix the Parmesan into the pasta and refrigerate it in a sealed container.

Southwestern Quinoa–Black Bean Salad

SERVES 4 (SERVING SIZE IS ABOUT 1¾ CUPS)

Calories per serving: 390

▸   SODIUM PER SERVING: 315 MG

Quinoa (pronounced Keen-wah) has pretty much everything you could want in a grain. High in fiber, quinoa is a complete protein, with all the protein components your body needs, and is a good source of calcium, magnesium, and iron. All that, and it's gluten-free, too! The small grains have a nutty flavor, similar to that of brown rice.

FOR THE DRESSING:

2 TABLESPOONS EXTRA-VIRGIN OLIVE OIL

1 TABLESPOON FRESHLY SQUEEZED LIME JUICE

¼ TEASPOON FRESHLY GROUND BLACK PEPPER

¼ TEASPOON GROUND CUMIN

¼ TEASPOON GROUND CORIANDER

½ CUP THINLY SLICED SCALLIONS

1 TABLESPOON CHOPPED FRESH PARSLEY

2 TABLESPOONS CHOPPED FRESH CILANTRO (OPTIONAL)

FOR THE SALAD:

½ CUP DRY QUINOA

1 (15-OUNCE) CAN LOW-SODIUM BLACK BEANS, DRAINED, RINSED, AND
     SHAKEN DRY

2 CUPS CHOPPED TOMATOES

1 RED BELL PEPPER, SEEDED AND CHOPPED

1 GREEN BELL PEPPER, SEEDED AND CHOPPED

2 TABLESPOONS MINCED JALAPEÑO PEPPERS (OPTIONAL)

To make the dressing:

1. In a small bowl, whisk together the oil, lime juice, pepper, cumin, and coriander.

2. Mix in the scallions, parsley, and cilantro (if using). Set aside.

To make the salad:

1. Cook the quinoa according to the directions on the package; then remove the pan from the heat and set it aside to cool for 15 minutes.

2. In a large bowl, mix the beans with the vegetables and jalapeño (if using). Add the cooled quinoa and stir everything together.

3. Pour the dressing over the salad and stir to coat.

4. Divide the salad into equal portions on 4 serving plates.

5. To save the salad for later, refrigerate it in a sealed container.

Bulgur and Chickpea Salad

SERVES 4 (SERVING SIZE IS ABOUT 1⅓ CUPS)

Calories per serving: 285

▸ SODIUM PER SERVING: 256 MG

Bulgur is a whole-wheat grain that has been cracked, partially cooked, and dried. It comes in various sizes, from fine to extra-coarse. With all the flavor, fiber, and nutrients of unrefined wheat, bulgur has a texture that will remind you of couscous. It is the main ingredient in tabbouleh and many other Middle Eastern dishes.

FOR THE DRESSING:

2 TABLESPOONS EXTRA-VIRGIN OLIVE OIL

3 TABLESPOONS FRESHLY SQUEEZED LEMON JUICE

¼ TEASPOON SALT

1 GARLIC CLOVE, MINCED

1 TABLESPOON MINCED FRESH PARSLEY

½ TEASPOON FRESHLY GROUND BLACK PEPPER

FOR THE SALAD:

1 CUP UNCOOKED COARSE BULGUR

¾ CUP CANNED CHICKPEAS, DRAINED, RINSED, AND SHAKEN DRY

½ CUP FINELY CHOPPED CARROTS

½ CUP RAISINS

½ CUP THINLY SLICED SCALLIONS

To make the dressing:

In a small bowl, whisk together all the ingredients. Set aside.

To make the salad:

1. Cook the bulgur according to the directions on the package, taking care that it does not become mushy. Remove it from the heat, fluff it with a fork, and set it aside to cool for 15 minutes.

2. In a medium bowl, mix together the cooled bulgur, chickpeas, carrots, raisins, and scallions.

3. Add the dressing and mix well.

4. Cover and chill the salad for at least 1 hour before serving.

5. Divide the salad into equal portions on 4 serving plates.

6. To save the salad for later, refrigerate it in a sealed container.

Creamy Butternut-Apple Soup

SERVES 4 (SERVING SIZE IS 1½ CUPS)

Calories per serving: 349

▶ SODIUM PER SERVING: 366 MG

Warm and naturally sweet, this soup isn't just for lunch. It's wonderful at any meal or as a snack. Autumn's glorious squash gives the soup the brilliant orange color of turning leaves, while the apples remind you of the fall harvest. Indeed, this soup is ideal on a blustery day. If you don't want your apple garnish to turn brown while you prepare the soup, toss the freshly grated apple with just a tiny bit of lemon juice.

1 (2½-POUND) BUTTERNUT SQUASH
2 TABLESPOONS EXTRA-VIRGIN OLIVE OIL
2 APPLES, PEELED, CORED, AND GRATED
1 CUP WATER
¼ TEASPOON GROUND CINNAMON
¼ TEASPOON GROUND DRY GINGER
¼ TEASPOON GROUND ALLSPICE
2 (12-OUNCE) CANS NONFAT EVAPORATED MILK
¼ TEASPOON SALT
⅛ TEASPOON FRESHLY GROUND BLACK PEPPER

1. Preheat the oven to 400°F.

2. Cut the squash in half lengthwise and scoop out and discard the seeds.

3. Brush the cut sides of the squash with 1 tablespoon of oil and place the halves on a baking sheet, cut side down. Bake until a sharp knife easily punctures the thickest part of the squash, 45 minutes to 1 hour.

4. Remove the squash from the oven and allow it to cool until it can be handled. Scoop the flesh out and discard the skins. Set the flesh aside.

5. In a large saucepan over medium heat, heat the remaining 1 tablespoon of oil. Add half the grated apple and cook until it softens, about 5 minutes.

6. Turn the heat up to medium-high, add the squash and water, and bring to a boil.

7. Turn the heat down to medium and simmer for 5 minutes.

8. Use a potato masher to mash the squash; then stir in the spices, evaporated milk, salt, and pepper.

9. Bring the soup back to a boil; then immediately remove it from the heat. Allow it to cool for 30 minutes.

10. Working in batches, ladle the soup into a blender and purée it until it is smooth. Return the puréed soup to the pot and heat it, stirring occasionally, over medium-low heat, until it is steaming.

11. Ladle the soup into 4 bowls and top each with the remaining apple.

12. To save the soup for later, refrigerate or freeze it in a sealed container or heavy plastic zip-top bag.

Turkey Noodle Soup

Calories per serving: 452

▸ SODIUM PER SERVING: 434 MG

Every year when Thanksgiving comes around, you most likely have one question on your mind: "What am I going to do with all this leftover turkey?" Make soup, of course! Thanks to the herbs and vegetables, this recipe delivers all the richness of your mom's homemade soup, with a lot less fat and sodium.

1 RIB CAGE FROM A COOKED TURKEY CARCASS, LEFTOVER BREAST
   MEAT ATTACHED
2 WHITE OR YELLOW ONIONS, CHOPPED
4 CELERY STALKS, SLICED CROSSWISE INTO ¼-INCH CRESCENTS
2 MEDIUM CARROTS, SLICED INTO ¼-INCH DISCS
WATER
2 CUPS CHOPPED BREAST MEAT FROM THE LEFTOVER COOKED TURKEY
1 TEASPOON DRIED SAGE
1 TEASPOON DRIED THYME
½ TEASPOON DRIED MARJORAM
½ TEASPOON DRIED ROSEMARY
½ TEASPOON SALT
½ TEASPOON FRESHLY GROUND BLACK PEPPER
8 OUNCES TINY DRY WHOLE-WHEAT PASTA SHAPES, SUCH AS ORZO,
   STELLINI (STARS), OR CONCHIGLIETTE (TINY SHELLS)

1. Put the turkey carcass, onions, celery, and carrots in a stockpot. Add water until the pot is about three-fourths full.

2. Over high heat, bring the water to a boil; then turn the heat down to medium-low and simmer, covered, for 2½ hours.

3. Remove the pot from the heat and transfer the vegetables to a bowl. Place the carcass on a cutting board. Set the turkey stock aside to cool for about 1 hour.

4. While the stock is cooling, pick any bits of meat off the ribs. If necessary, chop up the pieces.

5. When the stock is cool, skim the layer of fat off the top and discard. Pour the stock through a strainer and return it to the pot.

6. Add the picked meat and cooked vegetables back to the stock; then stir in the chopped meat, herbs, salt, and pepper.

7. Over medium-high heat, bring the soup to a low boil. Add the pasta and boil gently for 20 minutes.

8. Ladle the soup into bowls and serve piping hot.

9. To save the soup for later, refrigerate or freeze it in a sealed container or heavy plastic zip-top bag.

Traditional Beef Stew

SERVES 4 (SERVING SIZE IS 1½ CUPS)

Calories per serving: 319

▸ SODIUM PER SERVING: 607 MG

Yes, low-sodium, low-calorie foods really can stick to your ribs. This meat-and-potatoes dish is one of them. The rich flavors of the chunky stew make it even more sustaining.

2 TABLESPOONS WHOLE-WHEAT FLOUR

8 OUNCES TOP SIRLOIN STEAK, VISIBLE FAT TRIMMED, CUT INTO
    ¾-INCH CUBES

1 TABLESPOON EXTRA-VIRGIN OLIVE OIL

1 CUP LOW-SODIUM BEEF BROTH, DIVIDED

1 WHITE OR YELLOW ONION, CHOPPED

2 CARROTS, SLICED INTO ½-INCH DISCS

1 CELERY STALK WITH ITS LEAVES, DICED

1 POTATO, CUT INTO ¾-INCH CUBES

1 CUP SLICED BUTTON OR CREMINI MUSHROOMS

½ TEASPOON DRIED ROSEMARY

½ TEASPOON DRIED SAGE

½ TEASPOON DRIED TARRAGON

½ TEASPOON DRIED THYME

1 TEASPOON FRESHLY GROUND BLACK PEPPER

½ TEASPOON SALT

1 (14.5-OUNCE) CAN NO-SALT-ADDED DICED TOMATOES, WITH JUICE

2 TABLESPOONS ARROWROOT POWDER

¼ CUP 1 PERCENT MILK

1. Spread the flour out on a plate and dredge the steak on both sides to coat. Shake off excess flour and set the steak aside.

2. In a large saucepan over medium-high heat, heat the oil. Place the steak in the pan and brown it on all sides, about 2 minutes per side. Remove the meat.

3. Turn the heat down to medium. Pour ¼ cup of broth into the saucepan and deglaze the pan, scraping any brown bits off the bottom.

4. Add the onion, carrots, celery, potato, mushrooms, herbs, pepper, salt, and remaining ¾ cup of broth. Simmer for 15 minutes.

5. Add the browned steak and canned tomatoes. Simmer until the vegetables are cooked through but firm, about 10 minutes.

6. In a small bowl, stir the arrowroot into the milk until the mixture is smooth.

7. Add the arrowroot mixture to the saucepan, stir, and continue simmering until the stew thickens, about 5 minutes.

8. Spoon the stew into bowls and serve piping hot.

9. To save the stew for later, refrigerate or freeze it in a sealed container or heavy plastic zip-top bag.

Lentils and Kale over Brown Rice

SERVES 4 (SERVING SIZE IS ABOUT 2 CUPS)

Calories per serving: 456

▸ SODIUM PER SERVING: 328 MG

The savory, nutty, sweet layers of flavor in this dish make a lunch to look forward to. All but fat-free (except for a little olive oil), this tasty combo fills you with complex carbohydrates—the right kind of calories.

1 CUP UNCOOKED BROWN RICE

1 CUP UNCOOKED BROWN LENTILS

4 CUPS CHOPPED KALE, STEMS REMOVED

2 TABLESPOONS EXTRA-VIRGIN OLIVE OIL

1 WHITE OR YELLOW ONION, DICED

½ TEASPOON SALT

⅛ TEASPOON FRESHLY GROUND BLACK PEPPER

1. Cook the brown rice according to the directions on the package.

2. Cook the lentils according to the directions on the package.

3. About 15 minutes after the lentils start cooking, scatter the kale over them and cover the pot. Continue cooking until the lentils are tender but firm and the kale is tender, 5 to 10 minutes.

4. In a medium skillet over medium heat, heat the oil and add the onion, salt, and pepper. Cook, stirring often, until the onions are soft and deep brown but not burned, 10 to 15 minutes.

5. Stir the cooked lentils and kale into the pan with the caramelized onions.

6. Spoon one-fourth of the cooked rice onto each of 4 plates. Top each serving of rice with one-fourth of the lentil-kale mixture, and serve.

7. To save the dish for later, refrigerate it in a sealed container. Do not freeze.

Mini English Muffin Pizzas

Calories per serving: 240

▶   SODIUM PER SERVING: 365 MG

Almost everyone loves pizza. If you do, too, you'll enjoy these handy little treats. Serve these to your kids to get them DASHing!

1 CUP CANNED NO-SALT-ADDED TOMATO SAUCE

¼ TEASPOON DRIED BASIL

¼ TEASPOON DRIED OREGANO

1 CUP CHOPPED GREEN VEGETABLES, SUCH AS BROCCOLI, BELL PEPPERS, OR SPINACH

2 TO 3 TABLESPOONS WATER

4 WHOLE-WHEAT ENGLISH MUFFINS, HALVED AND TOASTED

½ CUP SHREDDED PART-SKIM MOZZARELLA CHEESE

3 TABLESPOONS SHREDDED CARROT

4 TEASPOONS GRATED PARMESAN CHEESE

1. Move the broiler pan to the lowest position and preheat the broiler.

2. In a small saucepan over medium heat, bring the tomato sauce to a simmer.

3. Add the basil and oregano and cook, covered, for 10 minutes.

4. In a small skillet over medium heat, simmer the green vegetables with the water until crisp-tender. Transfer the vegetables to paper towels to dry.

5. Spoon 2 tablespoons of tomato sauce over each toasted English muffin half.

6. Sprinkle 1 tablespoon of mozzarella over each muffin half.

7. Distribute the green vegetables and carrots equally over the muffins.

8. Sprinkle the top of each muffin with ½ teaspoon of Parmesan.

continued ▶

9. Put the muffin pizzas in the broiler and cook, monitoring carefully, until the cheese melts, 3 minutes or less.

10. Serve 2 pizzas on each plate and eat immediately.

11. To save the pizzas for later, let them cool completely. They will keep in the refrigerator, in a sealed container, for no more than 4 hours; longer than that and they will get soggy. Alternatively, wrap each cooled pizza in foil, put them together in a sealed container, and freeze. Chilled or frozen, the pizzas may be reheated in a toaster oven or microwave.

Tuna-Apple Salad Sandwiches

SERVES 4

Calories per serving: 270

▶ SODIUM PER SERVING: 231 MG

A lunchtime classic, tuna salad sandwiches have filled lunch boxes and brown bags for generations. This take replaces the mayonnaise with an herbed vinaigrette and adds some apple for crunch. It's great in a wrap, too.

FOR THE VINAIGRETTE:

2 TABLESPOONS EXTRA-VIRGIN OLIVE OIL

1 TABLESPOON RED WINE VINEGAR

1 TABLESPOON FRESHLY SQUEEZED LEMON JUICE

1 GARLIC CLOVE, MINCED

1 TEASPOON DRIED OREGANO

1 TEASPOON DRIED TARRAGON

¼ TEASPOON SALT

¼ TEASPOON FRESHLY GROUND BLACK PEPPER

FOR THE TUNA SALAD:

2 (6-OUNCE) CANS LOW-SODIUM CHUNK LIGHT TUNA PACKED
    IN WATER, DRAINED

2 TABLESPOONS MINCED RED ONION

1 APPLE, CORED AND CHOPPED

1 CUP CHOPPED CELERY

1 CUP GOLDEN RAISINS

FOR THE SANDWICHES:

2 CUPS MIXED SALAD GREENS

2 WHOLE-WHEAT PITA POCKETS, CUT IN HALF

continued ▶

To make the vinaigrette:

In a small bowl, whisk together all the ingredients. Set aside.

To make the tuna:

1. In a small bowl, break up the tuna with a fork.

2. Mix in the onion, apple, celery, raisins, and 2 tablespoons of vinaigrette. Set aside.

To make the sandwiches:

1. In a medium bowl, toss the salad greens with the remaining vinaigrette.

2. Fill each pita half with ¾ cup of the tuna and ½ cup of the greens, and serve.

3. To save the sandwiches for later, refrigerate the tuna, greens, and pitas separately in sealed containers. Do not freeze.

Fish Tacos

Calories per serving: 322

▸ SODIUM PER SERVING: 395 MG

The fresh tang of lime juice and the crispy crunch of cabbage complement the silky richness of the salmon in this Mexican-inspired dish. If you're looking for excitement, add a little extra heat with a few drops of hot sauce on top. Abundant in protein and fiber, each taco will keep your hunger in check for hours.

FOR THE MARINADE:

2 TEASPOONS EXTRA-VIRGIN OLIVE OIL

1 TABLESPOON FRESHLY SQUEEZED LIME JUICE

1 TABLESPOON CHILI POWDER

¼ TEASPOON SALT

FOR THE TACOS:

4 (3-OUNCE) SALMON FILLETS

1 CUP SHREDDED GREEN CABBAGE

1 RED ONION, QUARTERED AND THINLY SLICED INTO CRESCENTS

1 JALAPEÑO PEPPER, SEEDED AND MINCED

1 TEASPOON FINELY CHOPPED FRESH CILANTRO (OPTIONAL)

1 TABLESPOON FRESHLY SQUEEZED LIME JUICE

4 (8-INCH) WHOLE-WHEAT TORTILLAS

To make the marinade:

In a small bowl, whisk together all the ingredients.

To make the tacos:

1. Rinse the fish and pat it dry.

continued ▸

Fish Tacos *continued* ▶

2. In a medium bowl, pour the marinade over the salmon. Turn the fillets to thoroughly coat them.

3. Set the fish aside for 30 minutes. Every 5 minutes, flip the fillets over to marinate evenly.

4. Preheat the grill or broiler to high.

5. In another medium bowl, combine the cabbage, onion, jalapeño, cilantro (if using), and lime juice. Let the mixture rest for 15 minutes.

6. Place the salmon on the grill or in the broiler. Cook until the fish is flaky but still moist, 3 to 4 minutes on each side.

7. Transfer the fillets to a cutting board and allow them to rest for 3 minutes. Cut the fillets crosswise into ¼-inch slices.

8. Place each tortilla on a plate and lay 1 sliced fillet in the center. Top each with one-fourth of the cabbage mixture.

9. Eat the tacos with your hands (1 taco per serving), folding the tortilla in half around the filling.

10. To save the tacos for later, refrigerate the tortillas and filling separately in sealed containers. Do not freeze.

Chicken-Grape Salad Sandwiches

SERVES 5

Calories per serving: 289

▸ SODIUM PER SERVING: 350 MG

This recipe lends a little country club flair to an old standby. Add some variety by substituting chopped apple for the grapes, green bell peppers for the celery, or whole-wheat bread or a wrap for the rye bread. You may even add some chopped walnuts if you can afford the extra calories.

3¼ COOKED BONELESS, SKINLESS CHICKEN BREAST, CUBED
½ CUP QUARTERED SEEDLESS GREEN GRAPES
¼ CUP CHOPPED CELERY
¼ CUP THINLY SLICED SCALLIONS
1 TABLESPOON FRESHLY SQUEEZED LEMON JUICE
3 TABLESPOONS LIGHT MAYONNAISE
5 SLICES RYE BREAD
5 LEAVES ROMAINE LETTUCE

1. In a large bowl, mix together the chicken, grapes, celery, scallions, lemon juice, and mayonnaise.

2. Lightly toast the bread. Cut each slice in half.

3. Spread ¾ cup of the chicken mixture onto 1 half-slice of bread.

4. Tear up 1 lettuce leaf into large pieces and lay it over the chicken.

5. Top the lettuce with the other half-slice of bread.

6. Repeat for the rest of the sandwiches.

7. To save the sandwiches for later, refrigerate the chicken, lettuce, and untoasted bread separately in sealed containers. Do not freeze.

Chicken Quesadillas with Pico de Gallo

Calories per serving: 339

▶   SODIUM PER SERVING: 309 MG

Is there a more guilty pleasure than melted cheese? This dish gives you permission to indulge. Better yet, your kids will go for it, too. You may substitute parsley for the cilantro, if you like. And if you're not a fan of spicy dishes, swap regular Monterey jack cheese for the pepper jack and leave off the hot sauce.

FOR THE PICO DE GALLO:

2 CUPS DICED TOMATOES

½ CUP DICED RED ONION

1 JALAPEÑO PEPPER, SEEDED AND MINCED

2 TABLESPOONS FRESHLY SQUEEZED LIME JUICE

2 TABLESPOONS CHOPPED FRESH CILANTRO

1 TEASPOON GROUND CUMIN

FOR THE QUESADILLAS:

4 (10-INCH) WHOLE-WHEAT TORTILLAS

12 OUNCES COOKED BONELESS, SKINLESS CHICKEN BREAST, DICED

1 CUP SHREDDED PEPPER JACK CHEESE

½ TEASPOON HOT SAUCE (OPTIONAL)

To make the pico de gallo:

In a medium bowl, mix together all the ingredients. Cover and refrigerate for at least 1 hour and as long as 24 hours.

To make the quesadillas:

1. Preheat the oven to 350°F.

2. Lay a sheet of parchment paper or foil on a baking sheet.

3. In a medium skillet over medium-high heat, heat the tortillas one at a time until they brown slightly, about 1 minute per side. Place the tortillas on the baking sheet, evenly spaced.

4. Distribute the chicken evenly onto the 4 tortillas. Arrange it to cover half of each tortilla.

5. Scatter the cheese over the chicken, 2 tablespoons per tortilla.

6. Sprinkle hot sauce over the filling (if using).

7. Fold the empty half of each tortilla over the filled half and press down lightly.

8. Bake until the cheese is melted and the tortilla is golden brown, 8 to 10 minutes.

9. Transfer the quesadillas to a cutting board and cut each into 4 wedges.

10. Serve each quesadilla with ½ cup of pico de gallo on the side.

11. To save the quesadillas for later, allow them to cool completely; then refrigerate them in sealed containers. Alternately, wrap the cooled quesadillas separately in foil, put them together in a sealed container, and freeze. Chilled or frozen, the quesadillas may be reheated in a toaster oven or microwave.

Chicken-Lettuce Wraps with Spicy Soy Sauce

SERVES 4 (SERVING SIZE IS 2 WRAPS)

Calories per serving: 230

▸ SODIUM PER SERVING: 297 MG

An easy, high-heat cooking technique, stir-frying is traditionally done in a wok, whose curved interior lends itself to energetic tossing. You may use a large skillet instead, and the process will be just as fast, so have all your ingredients prepped and measured before you start cooking. Spice things up even more by adding a dash or two of hot sauce in the last thirty seconds of stir-frying.

FOR THE SAUCE:

1 JALAPEÑO PEPPER, SEEDED AND MINCED

2 GARLIC CLOVES, MINCED

1 TABLESPOON HONEY

2 TABLESPOONS FRESHLY SQUEEZED LIME JUICE

2 TEASPOONS LOW-SODIUM SOY SAUCE

½ CUP WATER

FOR THE CHICKEN:

12 OUNCES BONELESS, SKINLESS CHICKEN BREAST

1 TABLESPOON CANOLA OIL

2 GARLIC CLOVES, MINCED

1 TABLESPOON GRATED FRESH GINGER

½ CUP SHREDDED CARROT

1 TABLESPOON LOW-SODIUM SOY SAUCE

1 TABLESPOON SESAME OIL

1 TABLESPOON SESAME SEEDS

FOR THE WRAPS:

8 LARGE LEAVES BOSTON OR BUTTER LETTUCE

8 FRESH BASIL LEAVES

2 CUPS SHREDDED NAPA (ASIAN) OR SAVOY CABBAGE

To make the sauce:

1. In a small saucepan over high heat, combine all the ingredients and bring to a boil.

2. Remove the saucepan from the heat and allow the sauce to rest in the saucepan for 5 minutes.

3. Transfer the sauce to a heatproof container and refrigerate it until cold, at least 15 minutes.

To make the chicken:

1. Rinse the chicken and pat it dry. Cut the breasts crosswise into thin strips.

2. Heat a large skillet or wok over medium-high heat. Add the oil and heat it until it is hot but not smoking. Add the garlic and ginger. Stir-fry, stirring quickly and constantly, for 30 seconds to 1 minute.

3. Add the chicken and carrot and stir-fry for 5 or 6 minutes.

4. Add the soy sauce, sesame oil, and sesame seeds, stir well, and bring the liquid to a boil; then remove the chicken from the heat.

To make the wraps:

1. Place a lettuce leaf on a plate and top it with ½ cup of the chicken. Add 1 basil leaf and ¼ cup of the cabbage.

2. Repeat until you have made 8 wraps.

3. Arrange 2 wraps on each plate, and serve each plate with ¼ cup of the sauce.

4. To save the wraps for later, refrigerate the sauce, chicken, and lettuce separately in sealed containers. Do not freeze.

Swanky Steak Sandwiches

SERVES 4

Calories per serving: 321

▸   SODIUM PER SERVING: 391 MG

To make these elegant sandwiches as succulent as possible, it's essential to slice the steak against the grain. Take a look at any piece of red meat, and you'll see long fibers running through it in one general direction. These can make steak tough. But when you slice across the fibers—against the grain—you cut them. This gives you much more tender meat.

6 GARLIC CLOVES, IN THEIR SKINS
1 RED BELL PEPPER, SEEDED AND QUARTERED
1 YELLOW BELL PEPPER, SEEDED AND QUARTERED
2 TABLESPOONS EXTRA-VIRGIN OLIVE OIL
12 OUNCES TOP ROUND STEAK, VISIBLE FAT TRIMMED OFF
¼ TEASPOON FRESHLY GROUND BLACK PEPPER
8 SMALL (ABOUT 4-BY-5-INCH) SLICES OF CRUSTY, CHEWY, WHOLE-
    GRAIN BREAD
2 TABLESPOONS LIGHT MAYONNAISE
1 TABLESPOON DIJON MUSTARD
1 CUP MIXED BABY SALAD GREENS

1. Preheat the grill or broiler to medium-high.

2. In a medium bowl, toss the garlic and bell peppers with the oil.

3. Pick out the garlic cloves and place them on a piece of foil. Gather the edges together and pinch the foil closed to create a tight packet.

4. Put the garlic packet on the grill or under the broiler toward one side, so it receives indirect heat.

5. Put the bell peppers on the center of the grill or broiler pan. Cook the vegetables, turning the peppers occasionally, for 10 minutes. Transfer the garlic packet and vegetables to a cutting board and set aside to cool.

6. Sprinkle the steak all over with the black pepper. Broil or grill the meat until it reaches the desired temperature (about 4 minutes per side for medium-rare). Transfer the steak to a cutting board and let it rest for 5 minutes.

7. Put the bread on the grill or under the broiler and toast, turning once, until it is lightly browned, about 1 minute per side. Transfer the toast to a plate and set aside.

8. When the vegetables are cool enough to handle, cut the bell peppers into $\frac{1}{2}$-inch-wide strips.

9. Peel the garlic cloves and cut them into a few pieces.

10. In a small bowl, mash the garlic with any oil left in the foil packet. Add the mayonnaise and mustard and stir until well combined.

11. Thinly slice the steak against the grain.

12. Place a slice of toast on a plate and spread $1\frac{1}{2}$ teaspoons of the garlic mixture onto it. Put $\frac{1}{4}$ cup of the greens on the bread. Lay one-fourth of the red pepper and one-fourth of the yellow pepper on top of the greens. Top with one-fourth of the steak. Spread another slice of toast with $1\frac{1}{2}$ teaspoons of the garlic mixture and close the sandwich.

13. Repeat to make 3 more sandwiches.

14. To save the sandwiches for later, refrigerate the steak, spread, toast, and greens separately in sealed containers. Do not freeze.

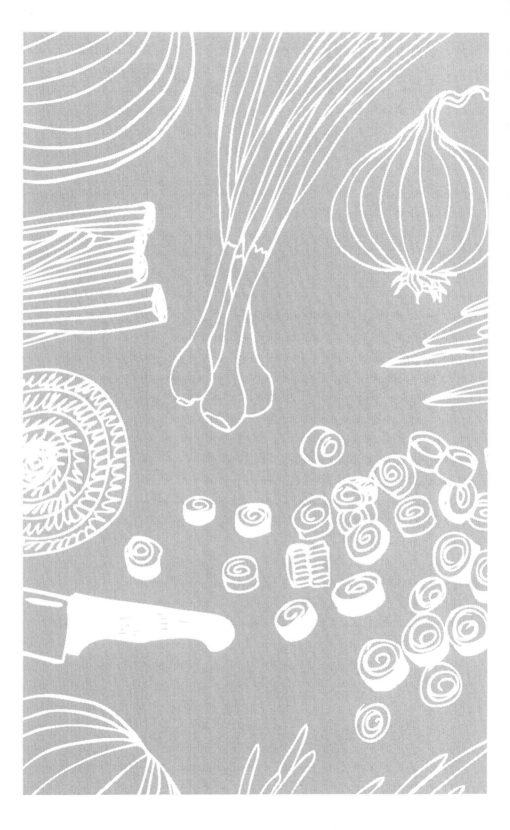

CHAPTER NINE

DASH Side Dishes

TUSCAN KALE SALAD MASSAGED WITH ROASTED GARLIC

PERFECT COLESLAW

SPANISH-STYLE SAUTÉED BABY SPINACH

LIMA BEANS WITH SPINACH

LEMONY ROASTED BROCCOLI

CINNAMON-ROASTED GLAZED CARROTS

PARMESAN-CRUSTED CAULIFLOWER

BLACK BEAN CONFETTI SALAD

BROWN RICE PILAF

ZESTY QUINOA

AROMATIC ALMOND COUSCOUS

PILAF PARMESAN

ASIAN NOODLES

MAPLE-PECAN MASHED SWEET POTATOES

JALAPEÑO CORNBREAD

Tuscan Kale Salad Massaged with Roasted Garlic

SERVES 4 (SERVING SIZE IS 1 CUP)

Calories per serving: 241

▸ SODIUM PER SERVING: 244 MG

Back in the day, restaurants and stores relegated kale to the role of decoration rather than food. Even though this leafy green is extremely good for you—it's absolutely packed with the antioxidant vitamins A, C, and K—it can be tough, so most customers weren't interested in eating it. Recently, though, kale has become increasingly popular as people have discovered how delicious it is when prepared properly. This salad uses Tuscan kale (also known as lacinato or dinosaur kale), rather than the more familiar curly variety because Tuscan kale is more tender, especially when raw.

FOR THE DRESSING:
1 HEAD GARLIC, WHOLE, UNPEELED BUT WITH LOOSE, PAPERY
   SKIN REMOVED
1 TABLESPOON PLUS 2½ TEASPOONS EXTRA-VIRGIN OLIVE OIL, DIVIDED
2 TABLESPOONS FRESHLY SQUEEZED LEMON JUICE
1 TABLESPOON LOW-SODIUM SOY SAUCE
½ TEASPOON FRESHLY GROUND BLACK PEPPER

FOR THE SALAD:
1 RED ONION, THINLY SLICED AND SEPARATED INTO RINGS
1 TABLESPOON EXTRA-VIRGIN OLIVE OIL
4 BUNCHES (ABOUT 1½ POUNDS) TUSCAN KALE
½ CUP UNSWEETENED DRIED CRANBERRIES
¼ CUP CHOPPED UNSALTED HAZELNUTS

To make the dressing:

1. Preheat the oven to 500°F.

2. Cut off the pointy end of the garlic head, so the tips of the cloves are sliced open.

3. Coat the outside of the whole head with ½ teaspoon of oil. Put the head on a piece of foil, gather the edges of the foil together, and pinch to create a tight packet.

4. Roast the garlic until it is very soft, about 45 minutes. Remove it from the oven and set aside to cool.

5. When the garlic is cool enough to handle, use your hands over a medium bowl to squeeze the head and push the garlic flesh out of its skin. Break the head apart and squeeze any cloves that still contain flesh.

6. Mash the flesh with the back of a spoon; then add the lemon juice, soy sauce, pepper, and remaining 1 tablespoon and 2 teaspoons of oil, and whisk until thoroughly combined.

To make the salad:

1. In a medium bowl, toss the onion rings with the oil. Spread the rings on a baking sheet.

2. When the garlic has roasted for 30 minutes, put the onions in the oven and roast, stirring once or twice, until the onions are soft and golden brown, about 15 minutes. Remove the onions from the oven and set aside to cool.

3. Cut the tough stem out of each kale leaf, about two-thirds of the way up the leaf.

4. Working in batches, roll together several leaves at a time like a cigar and cut crosswise to make ½-inch-wide strips. There should be about 6 cups of kale strips.

5. In a large bowl, toss the kale with the dressing. Use your hands to rub the dressing into the kale; it will soften and shrink slightly and turn a brighter green.

6. Add the cranberries, hazelnuts, and cooled onion, and toss to coat.

7. To save the salad for later, refrigerate it in a sealed container.

Perfect Coleslaw

Calories per serving: 93

▸ SODIUM PER SERVING: 236 MG

Crispy, creamy, and tangy, coleslaw is an ideal pairing for steaks, grilled chicken, and plain fish dishes, especially for Southern- and Southwestern-style recipes. Serve it on the side or add it to sandwiches. Because this version doesn't contain any eggs (in the form of mayonnaise) it keeps better, and more safely, than traditional coleslaw at summertime picnics.

¾ CUP NONFAT PLAIN GREEK YOGURT
2 TABLESPOONS DIJON MUSTARD
2 TABLESPOONS WHITE WINE VINEGAR
¼ TEASPOON SALT
½ TEASPOON CELERY SEEDS
4 CUPS SHREDDED GREEN CABBAGE
1 CUP SHREDDED RED CABBAGE
1 CUP SHREDDED CARROTS

1. In a large bowl, mix together the yogurt, mustard, vinegar, salt, and celery seeds.

2. Add the cabbages and carrots and toss to thoroughly coat.

3. Refrigerate, covered, for at least 1 hour to allow the flavors to blend before serving.

4. To save the coleslaw for later, refrigerate it in a sealed container.

Spanish-Style Sautéed Baby Spinach

SERVES 4 (SERVING SIZE IS 1 CUP)

Calories per serving: 136

▶ SODIUM PER SERVING: 180 MG

A traditional recipe from the Catalonia region of Spain, this is one of the most delicious ways to serve spinach. Its garlicky sweetness and tender crunchiness bring a lot of flavor to a plate of delicate fish and offer a pleasing contrast to dishes that contain tomato sauce. Add a dash of ground nutmeg for a more robust taste.

2 TABLESPOONS EXTRA-VIRGIN OLIVE OIL
3 GARLIC CLOVES, MINCED
20 OUNCES BABY SPINACH
WATER
⅔ CUP GOLDEN RAISINS
⅛ TEASPOON SALT
¼ CUP TOASTED PINE NUTS (PIGNOLI)

1. In a large skillet over medium heat, heat the oil. Add the garlic and sauté, stirring often, for 2 minutes, taking care not to brown the garlic.

2. Working in batches if necessary, add the spinach to almost fill the skillet. Add ¼ cup of water. Cook each batch until the spinach just begins to wilt, 1 to 2 minutes.

3. Move the wilted spinach to one side of the skillet. Add another batch of spinach; if the pan is dry, add another ¼ cup of water.

4. Repeat the process until all the spinach is in the skillet.

continued ▶

5. Turn the heat down to medium-low. If the skillet is dry, add 2 tablespoons of water. Stir in the raisins and salt. Cover the pan and steam for 3 minutes.

6. Uncover the skillet. Push the spinach to the side. If any liquid remains, turn the heat up to medium-high and cook until almost all the liquid evaporates.

7. Remove the skillet from the heat. Sprinkle the pine nuts over the spinach and toss to combine.

8. To save the spinach for later, allow it to cool completely, then refrigerate it in a sealed container.

Lima Beans with Spinach

Calories per serving: 93

▸ SODIUM PER SERVING: 362 MG

The butt of so many jokes, the lima bean is, for many people, the low legume on the bean pole. The canned type might deserve the ridicule, but the frozen variety deserves respect, and the fresh ones even more. Open your mind and try them again—or for the first time—and you'll discover the creamy richness that prompts some folks to call them butter beans. Limas are also awesome capsules of fiber, protein, magnesium, and vitamin C. Combine them with spinach, and you've got a delectable wallop of iron, too.

1 TABLESPOON EXTRA-VIRGIN OLIVE OIL
1 CUP CHOPPED FENNEL BULB, WITHOUT FRONDS
½ CUP CHOPPED WHITE OR YELLOW ONION
1 GARLIC CLOVE, MINCED
2 CUPS FROZEN OR FRESH LIMA BEANS, COOKED
¼ CUP WATER
10 OUNCES FRESH OR FROZEN SPINACH, CHOPPED
1 TABLESPOON CIDER VINEGAR
½ TEASPOON SALT
⅛ TEASPOON FRESHLY GROUND BLACK PEPPER

1. In a large skillet over medium heat, heat the oil and sauté the fennel, onion, and garlic until the onion and fennel are soft and golden brown.

2. Add the beans and water. Cook, covered, for 2 minutes.

3. Working in batches if necessary, add the spinach and cook until the leaves wilt, about 2 minutes.

4. Stir in the vinegar, salt, and pepper. Cook until the liquid almost entirely evaporates. Serve hot.

5. To save the dish for later, allow it to cool completely; then refrigerate it in a sealed container.

Lemony Roasted Broccoli

SERVES 4 (SERVING SIZE IS 1 CUP)

Calories per serving: 84

▸ SODIUM PER SERVING: 320 MG

Roasting in high, dry heat has a wonderful effect on most vegetables. As their moisture evaporates and their natural sugars caramelize, their flavors intensify and sweeten. If you're looking for an even deeper taste, toss in some sautéed, minced garlic when you add the lemon.

2 HEADS BROCCOLI, HEAVY STEMS REMOVED AND HEADS CUT INTO
  LARGE FLORETS
2 TABLESPOONS EXTRA-VIRGIN OLIVE OIL
½ TEASPOON SALT
¼ TEASPOON FRESHLY GROUND BLACK PEPPER
¼ CUP FRESHLY SQUEEZED LEMON JUICE
1 TEASPOON LEMON ZEST

1. Preheat the oven to 450°F.

2. In a large bowl, toss the broccoli with the oil, salt, and pepper.

3. Put the broccoli on a baking sheet and roast it until it is bright green and tender but not mushy, 10 to 12 minutes. It should have some crispy browned parts.

4. Transfer the broccoli back to the large bowl and toss it with the lemon juice and zest. Serve hot.

5. To save the broccoli for later, allow it to cool completely; then refrigerate it in a sealed container.

Cinnamon-Roasted Glazed Carrots

SERVES 4 (SERVING SIZE IS 3 TO 6 CARROTS)

Calories per serving: 42

▸ SODIUM PER SERVING: 124 MG

In this recipe, roasting concentrates the earthy sweetness of the carrots, and glazing enriches it with the dark flavor of brown sugar. Buy carrots with their tops still on; they are more tender and have softer skin, so they don't need peeling. You'll save time and also benefit from the precious nutrients in the skin. Leaving the carrots whole while roasting ensures that they won't dry out.

24 BABY CARROTS, TOPS CUT OFF AND DISCARDED
1 TABLESPOON EXTRA-VIRGIN OLIVE OIL
⅛ TEASPOON SALT
1 TABLESPOON SOFT TUB MARGARINE
2 TABLESPOONS PACKED DARK BROWN SUGAR
½ TEASPOON GROUND CINNAMON

1. Preheat the oven to 425°F.

2. Line a baking sheet with parchment paper or foil.

3. In a large bowl, toss the carrots with the oil and salt to coat.

4. Put the carrots on the baking sheet. Roast the carrots for 15 minutes; then remove them from the oven.

5. In a small saucepan over medium-low heat, melt the margarine. Stir in the brown sugar and cinnamon. Continue stirring until most of the sugar dissolves. Remove the pot from the heat.

continued ▸

6. Transfer the carrots to a large bowl. Leave the oiled paper or foil on the baking sheet.

7. Add the margarine mixture to the bowl with the carrots and toss to coat.

8. Put the carrots back on the baking sheet and drizzle them with any glaze left in the bowl.

9. Roast the carrots until they are tender but not soft, about 15 minutes. Serve hot.

10. To save the carrots for later, allow them to cool completely; then refrigerate them in a sealed container.

Parmesan-Crusted Cauliflower

Calories per serving: 60

▶   SODIUM PER SERVING: 209 MG

Who can resist sweet cauliflower with a crunchy, cheesy crust? And cauliflower will give you a big wallop of vitamin C, manganese, beta-carotene, and fiber.

1 HEAD CAULIFLOWER, LARGE STEMS REMOVED, CUT INTO FLORETS
1 TABLESPOON SOFT TUB MARGARINE
2 TABLESPOONS NO-SALT-ADDED WHOLE-WHEAT BREAD CRUMBS
⅛ TEASPOON FRESHLY GROUND BLACK PEPPER
⅛ TEASPOON SALT
1 TABLESPOON GRATED PARMESAN CHEESE
1 TABLESPOON CHOPPED FRESH PARSLEY
½ TEASPOON EXTRA-VIRGIN OLIVE OIL

1. Preheat the oven to 350°F.

2. Insert a steamer basket into a large saucepan and add 1 inch of water. Put the cauliflower in the steamer basket and cover the pot. Over medium-high heat, bring the water to a boil.

3. Turn the heat down to low and steam the cauliflower until it is crisp-tender, about 5 minutes. Transfer the cauliflower to a large bowl.

4. In a small saucepan over medium heat, melt the margarine.

5. Add the breadcrumbs, pepper, and salt. Stir and cook for 5 minutes.

6. Remove the pan from the heat and stir in the Parmesan and parsley.

7. Add the breadcrumb mixture to the bowl with the cauliflower and toss to coat.

continued ▶

8. Use the oil to grease the bottom and sides of a 9-by-9-inch baking dish. Put the cauliflower in the dish in an even layer.

9. Roast the cauliflower until the top is golden brown, about 25 minutes. Serve hot.

10. To save the cauliflower for later, allow it to cool completely; then refrigerate it in a sealed container.

Black Bean Confetti Salad

Calories per serving: 214

▶   SODIUM PER SERVING: 176 MG

Inspired by the flavors of the Southwest, this filling salad is great alongside grilled meat, chicken, or fish. It calls for frozen corn rather than canned corn kernels because the texture and flavor are far superior. If corn is in season and you've got the time and skill to prepare fresh corn kernels (you'll need two ears of corn), the results will be even better.

1 (15-OUNCE) CAN LOW-SODIUM BLACK BEANS, DRAINED AND RINSED

1 RED BELL PEPPER, SEEDED AND DICED

¾ CUP FROZEN CORN KERNELS, THAWED

½ CUP DICED RED ONION

1 JALAPEÑO PEPPER, SEEDED AND MINCED

2 TABLESPOONS CHOPPED FRESH CILANTRO

2 TABLESPOONS FRESHLY SQUEEZED LIME JUICE

2 TABLESPOONS CIDER VINEGAR

1 TABLESPOON EXTRA-VIRGIN OLIVE OIL

1 TEASPOON MINCED GARLIC

1. In a large bowl, combine all the ingredients.

2. Cover and refrigerate the salad for at least 1 hour to allow the flavors to marry before serving.

3. To save the salad for later, refrigerate it in a sealed container.

Brown Rice Pilaf

Calories per serving: 251

▸   SODIUM PER SERVING: 178 MG

The nutty flavor and slightly chewy texture of brown rice give this dish a bold character that's lacking in many white-rice pilafs. With the addition of lemon juice, it takes on a delightful brightness. If you want even more flavor, use low-sodium chicken broth in place of the water.

2 TEASPOONS EXTRA-VIRGIN OLIVE OIL
1½ CUPS FINELY CHOPPED WHITE OR YELLOW ONION
1¼ CUPS FINELY CHOPPED CELERY, WITH LEAVES
1 CUP UNCOOKED BROWN RICE
2½ CUPS WATER
2 TABLESPOONS FRESHLY SQUEEZED LEMON JUICE
¼ TEASPOON SALT
¼ CUP SLIVERED ALMONDS

1. In a large saucepan over medium heat, heat the oil. Add the onion and celery and cook until golden, about 5 minutes.

2. Add the rice, stir to coat, and cook for 1 minute.

3. Add the water, lemon juice, and salt. Turn the heat up to high and bring the liquid to a boil.

4. Reduce the heat to low and simmer, covered, for 30 minutes; then start checking the rice for doneness every 5 minutes. If the pot is dry before the rice is tender, add 2 tablespoons of water. The rice should be tender and most of the liquid should be absorbed within 40 to 50 minutes.

5. Remove the rice from the heat and let it stand, covered, for 5 minutes to absorb the rest of the liquid.

6. Fluff the rice with a fork and stir in the almonds. Serve hot.

7. To save the rice for later, allow it to cool completely; then refrigerate it in a sealed container.

Zesty Quinoa

Calories per serving: 117

▸   SODIUM PER SERVING: 103 MG

Before you cook quinoa, it's essential to rinse it. Quinoa is naturally coated with a bitter, soapy-tasting substance called saponin, which you'll want to remove to make the grain deliciously edible. Even if the package label says the quinoa is pre-rinsed, give it another rinse just to be sure.

1 CUP DRY QUINOA
1 TEASPOON EXTRA-VIRGIN OLIVE OIL
2 CUPS WATER
¼ TEASPOON SALT
½ TEASPOON PAPRIKA
¼ TEASPOON GROUND CUMIN
1 TABLESPOON CHOPPED FRESH CILANTRO

1. Put the quinoa in a large, fine-mesh strainer, and rinse it for 2 minutes under cool running water while swirling the quinoa around with your hand. Turn off the water and gently shake the sieve to remove as much water as possible.

2. In a medium saucepan over medium-high heat, heat the oil and add the quinoa. Stir for about 1 minute to dry and toast the quinoa.

3. Add the water, salt, paprika, and cumin. Bring the water to a boil. Turn the heat down to low, cover the pot, and cook until all of the water is absorbed, 10 to 15 minutes.

4. Remove the pot from the heat, stir in the cilantro, and let the quinoa stand, covered, for 5 minutes.

5. Fluff the quinoa with a fork before serving.

6. To save the quinoa for later, allow it to cool completely; then refrigerate it in a sealed container.

Aromatic Almond Couscous

SERVES 4 (SERVING SIZE IS ¾ CUP)

Calories per serving: 269

▶   SODIUM PER SERVING: 99 MG

Although it's cooked and used like a grain, couscous is actually a pasta. It is a signature ingredient in the cuisine of North Africa, where it's served with gently spiced stews of vegetables, meat (especially lamb), and dried fruit. The cinnamon and almonds in this recipe are customary North African flavors, but feel free to experiment with other spices or nuts.

2 TABLESPOONS EXTRA-VIRGIN OLIVE OIL
1 WHITE OR YELLOW ONION, CHOPPED
1½ CUPS LOW-SODIUM CHICKEN OR VEGETABLE BROTH
½ TEASPOON SALT
¼ TEASPOON GROUND CINNAMON
1 CUP WHOLE-WHEAT INSTANT COUSCOUS
¼ CUP SLIVERED ALMONDS
¼ CUP CHOPPED FRESH PARSLEY

1. In a large saucepan over medium-low heat, heat the oil and add the onion. Cook the onion until it is softened and golden, about 10 minutes.

2. Add the broth, salt, and cinnamon and bring to a boil.

3. Remove the pot from the heat and stir in the couscous. Cover the pot tightly and set it aside for 10 minutes. The couscous is done when it is tender but not mushy. If it's not soft enough, put the cover back on the pot for another 2 to 3 minutes.

4. Add the almonds and parsley and fluff the ingredients with a fork. Serve warm.

5. To save the couscous for later, allow it to cool completely; then refrigerate it in a sealed container.

Pilaf Parmesan

SERVES 6 (SERVING SIZE IS ⅔ CUP)

Calories per serving: 208

▸   SODIUM PER SERVING: 317 MG

It might seem redundant to use rice and pasta in the same dish, but it's done in the traditional cuisine of many countries, from Mexico to Greece. If you've ever had Rice-A-Roni, you've had a version that originated (yes, in San Francisco) as an Italian-Armenian hybrid. Although white rice is on the DASH diet list of foods to avoid, it's used in this recipe for flavor and texture and because it cooks more quickly than brown rice, making for a better pilaf.

2 TABLESPOONS EXTRA-VIRGIN OLIVE OIL

1 TABLESPOON MINCED WHITE OR YELLOW ONION

2 GARLIC CLOVES, MINCED

½ CUP BROKEN-UP, UNCOOKED, WHOLE-WHEAT VERMICELLI, ANGEL HAIR PASTA, OR MEXICAN FIDEO NOODLES

1 CUP UNCOOKED, LONG-GRAIN WHITE RICE

1 TEASPOON DRIED OREGANO

½ TEASPOON SALT

¼ TEASPOON FRESHLY GROUND BLACK PEPPER

1½ CUPS HOT CHICKEN BROTH

1½ CUPS HOT WATER

2 TABLESPOONS GRATED PARMESAN CHEESE

1. In a large skillet over medium-high heat, heat the oil. Add the onion and garlic and sauté for 1 minute.

2. Add the noodles and rice and cook until the noodles are golden brown, 2 to 4 minutes. Drain off the oil and discard.

3. Return the skillet to the heat and stir in the oregano, salt, and pepper.

4. Carefully pour in the broth and water (they may spatter if added too quickly).

5. Bring the liquid to a boil, turn the heat down to low, and cover the pan. Simmer until the noodles and rice are soft but not mushy, 15 to 20 minutes.

6. Remove the pilaf from the heat and let it stand, covered, for 5 minutes.

7. Add the Parmesan and fluff the pilaf with a fork to combine. Serve hot.

8. To save the pilaf for later, allow it to cool completely; then refrigerate it in a sealed container.

Asian Noodles

Calories per serving: 277

▸ SODIUM PER SERVING: 282 MG

Cool, tangy, and light, this dish is perfect on a summer evening or alongside any spicy or rich Asian-style dish. The brown rice noodles have more body than the white rice version, and some people find them easier to handle. If you want to add another flavor and texture, try sesame seeds or crushed peanuts.

FOR THE DRESSING:
¼ CUP FRESHLY SQUEEZED LIME JUICE
¼ CUP RICE VINEGAR
2 TEASPOONS SESAME OIL
1 TABLESPOON HONEY
¼ CUP CHOPPED FRESH CILANTRO
2 TEASPOONS GRATED FRESH GINGER
2 GARLIC CLOVES, MINCED
1 TEASPOON CRUSHED RED PEPPER FLAKES
⅛ TEASPOON SALT

FOR THE SALAD:
8 OUNCES UNCOOKED ASIAN BROWN RICE VERMICELLI
1 CARROT, GRATED
1 SCALLION, THINLY SLICED
½ CUCUMBER, PEELED AND GRATED

To make the dressing:

In a small bowl, whisk together all the ingredients. Set aside.

To make the salad:

1. Fill a large bowl two-thirds full with cold water and 1 tray of ice cubes.

2. Cook the noodles according to the directions on the package, with no salt added. When they are cooked and drained, transfer them to the ice water to cool completely. Drain well.

3. In a large bowl, toss the noodles with the dressing, carrot, scallion, and cucumber. Serve immediately.

4. To save the noodles for later, refrigerate them in a sealed container.

Maple-Pecan Mashed Sweet Potatoes

SERVES 4 (SERVING SIZE IS ½ CUP)

Calories per serving: 211

▸ SODIUM PER SERVING: 179 MG

Sweet potatoes have been called a superfood, and rightfully so. They're packed with fiber, vitamins A and C, and beta-carotene, to name only a few of their nutrients. Better yet, they taste fantastic! They even smell great while they're cooking.

1 OUNCE (ABOUT 20 HALVES) PECANS
2 LARGE SWEET POTATOES
6 TABLESPOONS PURE MAPLE SYRUP
¼ TEASPOON GROUND CINNAMON
¼ TEASPOON GROUND GINGER
¼ TEASPOON SALT

1. Preheat the oven to 375°F.

2. Spread the pecans out in a single layer on a baking sheet. Roast them until they are fragrant and slightly darker in color, about 5 minutes.

3. Remove the pecans from the oven and allow them to cool. When they can be handled, chop the nuts; there should be about ¼ cup.

4. Increase the oven heat to 400°F.

5. Use a fork to poke several small holes in the skin of each potato and place them directly on the oven rack. Bake until the potatoes are fork tender, 30 to 35 minutes. Let the potatoes cool until they can be handled.

6. In a small saucepan over medium heat, combine the syrup, cinnamon, and ginger. Bring to a gentle simmer. Remove the syrup from the heat and let it stand for about 5 minutes.

7. Scoop the flesh out of the cooked potatoes and put it in a medium microwave-safe bowl. Add the salt and mash the potato until it is smooth.

8. Mix in the syrup and the nuts.

9. To warm, microwave the potatoes on high for 3 minutes before serving.

10. To save the potatoes for later, allow them to cool completely; then refrigerate them in a sealed container.

Jalapeño Cornbread

SERVES 9 (SERVING SIZE IS 1 PIECE)

Calories per serving: 181

▶   SODIUM PER SERVING: 103 MG

Full of fiber and iron, and low in fat and sugar, this moist, sweet version proves that scrumptious cornbread doesn't have to be bad for you. Make it with a fine grind of cornmeal if you like a smooth texture or a coarser grind if you like a crunchier texture. Feel free to leave out the jalapeño if you want the sweet without the heat.

1½ CUPS CORNMEAL

½ CUP UNBLEACHED ALL-PURPOSE FLOUR

2 TABLESPOONS SUGAR

1 TEASPOON BAKING POWDER

1 EGG WHITE

1 CUP 1 PERCENT BUTTERMILK

¼ CUP SOFT TUB MARGARINE, MELTED

1 JALAPEÑO, SEEDED AND MINCED

1 TEASPOON CANOLA OIL

1. Preheat the oven to 350°F.

2. In a large bowl, mix together the cornmeal, flour, sugar, and baking powder.

3. In a small bowl, beat the egg white and stir in the buttermilk.

4. Mixing with a large spoon, add the buttermilk mixture to the dry ingredients. Stir in the margarine and the jalapeño.

5. Use the oil to grease the bottom and sides of an 8-by-8-inch baking dish. Pour in the batter and spread it evenly.

6. Bake the cornbread until the edges start to brown and a toothpick inserted in the center of the bread comes out clean, 20 to 25 minutes.

7. Transfer the dish to a wire rack and allow the bread to cool. To serve, cut the bread into 9 squares.

8. To save the cornbread for later, allow it to cool completely; then cover the baking dish tightly with plastic wrap and refrigerate. Alternately, wrap the cornbread in wax paper, put it in a tightly sealed container, and freeze it.

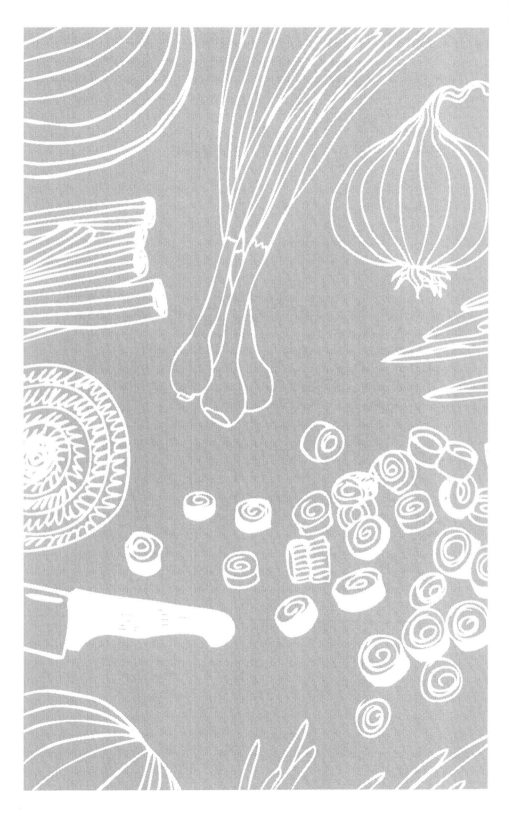

CHAPTER TEN

DASH Dinners

Green Lasagna

SERVES 8 (SERVING SIZE IS 1 PIECE)

Calories per serving: 185

▶ SODIUM PER SERVING: 310 MG

Who doesn't love lasagna? Hot, bubbling, cheese on top of ribbons of pasta, with zesty tomato sauce—what could be better? To guarantee this version is as tasty as can be, keep it from getting watery by pressing the moisture out of the zucchini.

1 LARGE ZUCCHINI, CUT INTO ¼-INCH SLICES

3 TEASPOONS EXTRA-VIRGIN OLIVE OIL

¼ CUP CHOPPED WHITE OR YELLOW ONION

2 GARLIC CLOVES, CHOPPED

2½ CUPS NO-SALT-ADDED TOMATO SAUCE

2 TEASPOONS DRIED BASIL

2 TEASPOONS DRIED OREGANO

⅛ TEASPOON FRESHLY GROUND BLACK PEPPER

¾ CUP PART-SKIM SHREDDED MOZZARELLA CHEESE, DIVIDED

4 TABLESPOONS GRATED PARMESAN CHEESE

1½ CUPS LOW-SODIUM NONFAT COTTAGE CHEESE

12 OUNCES WHOLE-WHEAT LASAGNA NOODLES, COOKED ACCORDING TO
    THE DIRECTIONS ON THE PACKAGE, NO SALT ADDED

1. On a clean tea towel or a double layer of paper towels laid out on a flat work surface, arrange the zucchini slices in a single layer. Place a layer of toweling over the zucchini. Put a large baking sheet on top, cooking side up, and distribute a few heavy objects (such as cans of food) evenly around the sheet. Let the weight press the moisture out of the zucchini until you are ready to use it, at least 30 minutes.

2. Preheat the oven to 350°F.

3. Use 1 teaspoon of the oil to grease the bottom and sides of a 9-by-13-inch baking pan.

4. In a medium saucepan over medium heat, heat the remaining 2 teaspoons of oil. Add the onion and garlic and cook, stirring occasionally, until the onion softens, about 5 minutes.

5. Add the tomato sauce, basil, oregano, and pepper, and stir to combine. Simmer for 20 minutes. Remove the sauce from the heat and set aside.

6. In a medium bowl, mix together 1/2 cup of mozzarella, 3 tablespoons of the Parmesan, and the cottage cheese. Set aside.

7. In a small bowl, mix together the remaining 1/4 cup of mozzarella and 1 tablespoon of Parmesan. Set aside.

8. Spread a thin layer (about 1/2 cup) of the tomato sauce over the bottom of the baking dish.

9. Lay 4 cooked lasagna noodles across the bottom of the pan to cover it.

10. Spoon half of the cottage cheese mixture onto the noodles, distributing it evenly.

11. Arrange half of the zucchini slices on top.

12. Repeat with a second layer of sauce, noodles, cheese, and zucchini.

13. Lay the remaining noodles over the top.

14. Spread on the remaining sauce, and sprinkle with the reserved mozzarella-Parmesan mixture.

15. Cover the lasagna with foil and bake for 30 minutes.

16. Remove the foil and bake the lasagna until the cheese on top bubbles and starts to brown, 10 to 15 minutes.

17. Remove the lasagna from the oven and let it stand for 15 minutes before cutting it into 8 pieces. Serve hot.

18. To save the lasagna for later, allow it to cool completely; then cover the pan tightly with foil and refrigerate or freeze. You may also freeze individual pieces: Wrap each piece tightly in foil and then store it in a heavy zip-top bag in the freezer.

Three-Bean Chili

SERVES 6 (SERVING SIZE IS 1½ CUPS)

Calories per serving: 331

▸ SODIUM PER SERVING: 469 MG

Chunky and well-seasoned, this hearty vegetarian chili will satisfy even hard-core carnivores. If you want to up the Tex-Mex quotient, stir in a tablespoon or two of chopped fresh cilantro at the end, and serve the chili with a splash of hot sauce. For tamer palates, substitute ground coriander for the chili powder.

2 TABLESPOONS EXTRA-VIRGIN OLIVE OIL

1 CUP COARSELY CHOPPED WHITE OR YELLOW ONION

1 TABLESPOON MINCED GARLIC

1 CUP SEEDED AND DICED GREEN BELL PEPPER

1 JALAPEÑO PEPPER, SEEDED AND MINCED (OPTIONAL)

1 (15-OUNCE) CAN LOW-SODIUM BLACK BEANS, DRAINED AND RINSED

1 (15-OUNCE) CAN LOW-SODIUM RED KIDNEY BEANS, DRAINED
    AND RINSED

1 (15-OUNCE) CAN LOW-SODIUM PINTO BEANS, DRAINED AND RINSED

1 (28-OUNCE) CAN NO-SALT-ADDED DICED TOMATOES

2 TABLESPOONS DRIED OREGANO

1 TABLESPOON DRIED BASIL

1 TABLESPOON GROUND CUMIN

1 TABLESPOON CHILI POWDER

¾ TEASPOON SALT

1. In a large saucepan over medium heat, heat the oil. Add the onion and garlic and cook, stirring occasionally, until the onion softens, about 5 minutes.

2. Add the green pepper and jalapeño (if using) and cook, stirring occasionally, until the peppers soften slightly, about 5 minutes.

3. Stir in the beans, tomatoes, oregano, basil, cumin, chili powder, and salt.

4. Turn the heat up to medium-high and bring the liquid to a boil. Turn the heat down to medium-low, cover the pot, and simmer for 20 minutes. Serve hot.

5. To save the chili for later, allow it to cool completely; then refrigerate or freeze it in a tightly sealed container.

Comforting Mac and Cheese

SERVES 6 (SERVING SIZE IS 1½ CUPS)

Calories per serving: 353

▸ SODIUM PER SERVING: 192 MG

You'll feel like a kid again when you dig into this mac and cheese, and your kids will be glad to join you. If you have a favorite cheese that's a good melter, you may swap it for some or all of the cheddar. Or get creative and make a complete one-dish meal by adding precooked chicken breast or vegetables such as peas, mushrooms, bell peppers, or broccoli.

2 CUPS DRY WHOLE-WHEAT MACARONI

1 TEASPOON CANOLA OIL

1 EGG, LIGHTLY BEATEN

½ CUP NONFAT EVAPORATED MILK

1¼ CUPS FINELY SHREDDED LOW-FAT SHARP CHEDDAR CHEESE

¼ TEASPOON DRY MUSTARD

⅛ TEASPOON FRESHLY GROUND BLACK PEPPER

¼ CUP NO-SALT-ADDED WHOLE-WHEAT BREAD CRUMBS

1. Preheat the oven to 350°F.

2. Cook the macaroni al dente, according to the directions on the package, with no salt added.

3. Use the oil to grease the bottom and sides of a 9-by-9-inch baking dish.

4. In a large bowl, combine the egg, milk, cheese, mustard, and pepper. Add the macaroni and stir to coat.

5. Pour the macaroni mixture into the baking dish. Sprinkle the bread crumbs on top.

6. Bake the macaroni until the bread crumbs are golden and the cheese is bubbly, about 25 minutes.

7. Remove the macaroni from the oven and allow it to stand for 10 minutes before serving.

8. To save the dish for later, allow it to cool completely; then refrigerate or freeze it in a tightly sealed container.

Creamy Sole with Grapes

SERVES 4 (SERVING SIZE IS 1 FILLET)

Calories per serving: 171

▶ SODIUM PER SERVING: 193 MG

Most fish is delicious in a light, tangy, cream sauce. In this recipe, you may use fillets from any variety of sole or from similar white-fleshed flatfish, such as halibut, flounder, or turbot. If you want to leave out the wine, add 2 more table-spoons of lemon juice.

4 (3-OUNCE) SOLE FILLETS

½ TEASPOON EXTRA-VIRGIN OLIVE OIL

¼ TEASPOON SALT

⅛ TEASPOON FRESHLY GROUND BLACK PEPPER

¼ CUP DRY WHITE WINE

¼ CUP LOW-SODIUM CHICKEN BROTH

1 TABLESPOON FRESHLY SQUEEZED LEMON JUICE

½ TEASPOON CHOPPED FRESH THYME

1 TABLESPOON SOFT TUB MARGARINE

2 TABLESPOONS UNBLEACHED ALL-PURPOSE FLOUR

¾ CUP 1 PERCENT MILK

½ CUP HALVED SEEDLESS GREEN GRAPES

1. Preheat the oven to 350°F.

2. Rinse the fish and pat it dry.

3. Use the oil to grease the bottom of an 11-by-7-inch baking dish. Place the fillets in the dish, and sprinkle them with the salt and pepper.

4. In a small bowl, combine the wine, chicken broth, lemon juice, and thyme. Pour the liquid over the fish.

5. Cover the dish with foil and bake the fish for 15 minutes.

6. In a small saucepan over low heat, melt the margarine.

7. Remove the pan from the heat and whisk in the flour until smooth.

8. Continue whisking and slowly pour in the milk.

9. Put the pan back on the stove over medium-low heat. Cook, whisking constantly, until the sauce thickens, about 5 minutes.

10. Remove the fish from the oven and transfer the fillets to a plate.

11. Preheat the broiler.

12. Position the broiler pan about 3 inches below the heating element.

13. Pour the liquid from the baking dish into the pan with the sauce and stir until thoroughly combined.

14. Return the fish to the baking dish and pour on the sauce. Scatter the grapes over the top.

15. Broil the fish until the sauce starts to brown, 5 minutes or less.

16. Transfer 1 fillet to each of 4 dinner plates. Spoon the sauce from the pan over the top of the fish. Serve immediately.

17. To save the fish for later, allow it to cool completely; then refrigerate it in a sealed container. Do not freeze.

Teriyaki Salmon Stir-Fry

Calories per serving: 274

▸ SODIUM PER SERVING: 389 MG

The mirin called for in this Japanese-style recipe is a sweet, golden rice wine made for cooking. It lends a delicate sweetness to dishes and makes glossy sauces that coat food well. If you can't find mirin, you may substitute a mixture of white sugar and white wine, dry sherry, or sake in a one-to-four ratio.

FOR THE SALMON:

1 TEASPOON CANOLA OIL

4 (3-OUNCE) SALMON FILLETS

¼ CUP MIRIN

2 TABLESPOONS RICE VINEGAR

1 TABLESPOON LOW-SODIUM SOY SAUCE

1 TABLESPOON HONEY

1 TABLESPOON MINCED GARLIC

1½ TABLESPOONS GRATED FRESH GINGER

FOR THE STIR-FRY:

2 TEASPOONS CANOLA OIL

1 TABLESPOON MINCED GARLIC

1 TABLESPOON MINCED FRESH GINGER

1 TABLESPOON THINLY SLICED SCALLION

1 CUP THINLY SLICED CARROTS

1 CUP SNAP PEAS OR SNOW PEAS, STRINGS REMOVED

1 CUP THINLY SLICED YELLOW SQUASH

1 CUP MUNG BEAN SPROUTS

1 TABLESPOON LOW-SODIUM SOY SAUCE

To make the salmon:

1. Preheat the oven to 350°F.

2. Grease a baking sheet with the oil.

3. Rinse the fish and pat it dry.

4. In a large bowl, whisk together the mirin, vinegar, soy sauce, honey, garlic, and ginger.

5. Add the salmon to the mixture and turn over the fillets several times to coat them.

6. Marinate the fillets for 10 minutes, turn over the fillets, and marinate them for 5 minutes more.

7. Transfer the salmon to the baking sheet and discard the leftover marinade.

8. Bake the fillets until the thickest fillet is not quite cooked through, 10 to 15 minutes.

9. Remove the fillets from the oven and cover lightly with foil to keep the fish warm.

To make the stir-fry:

1. Heat a large skillet or wok over medium-high heat. Add the oil and heat it until it is hot but not smoking.

2. Add the garlic, ginger, and scallions. Stir-fry, stirring quickly and constantly, for 30 seconds to 1 minute.

3. Add the carrots and snap peas, and stir-fry until the vegetables are crisp-tender, 2 to 3 minutes.

4. Add the squash and sprouts and continue to stir-fry until the squash is tender but not mushy, 1 to 2 minutes.

5. Add the soy sauce and toss the vegetables to coat. Remove the vegetables from the heat.

6. Dividing the vegetables evenly between 4 plates, arrange the vegetables in a mound. Place the salmon fillets on top. Serve immediately.

7. To save the dish for later, do not combine the salmon and vegetables. Allow each to cool completely; then refrigerate them in separate sealed containers. Do not freeze.

Oven-Fried Catfish

Calories per serving: 164

▸ SODIUM PER SERVING: 273 MG

This Southern-style dish gets its crunch from Japanese bread crumbs called panko. Once hard to find, they're now made by American as well as Japanese producers and are readily available in your supermarket. Panko is significantly lower in sodium than regular store-bought bread crumbs.

6 (5-OUNCE) CATFISH FILLETS
1 TABLESPOON FRESHLY SQUEEZED LEMON JUICE
¼ CUP 1 PERCENT BUTTERMILK
1 TEASPOON MINCED GARLIC
½ CUP PANKO BREAD CRUMBS
¼ TEASPOON GROUND CAYENNE PEPPER (OPTIONAL)
¼ TEASPOON FRESHLY GROUND BLACK PEPPER
¼ TEASPOON SALT
1 LEMON, CUT INTO 6 WEDGES

1. Preheat the oven to 475°F.

2. Place a wire rack in a roasting pan.

3. Rinse the fish and pat it dry.

4. Gently massage the lemon juice into the fillets and pat them dry.

5. In a wide, shallow bowl or pan, mix together the buttermilk and garlic.

6. Put the fillets in the bowl, turn them several times to coat, and gently massage the marinade into the fish. Set aside for 10 minutes.

7. In a small bowl, combine the panko, cayenne, black pepper, and salt. Transfer the mixture to a shallow dish.

8. Using your fingers, remove each fillet from the marinade, shake off the excess liquid, and dredge it in the panko mixture to coat both sides. Shake off any excess coating.

9. Put the dredged fillets on a plate and pat them lightly so the breading sticks to the fish.

10. Carefully transfer the fish to the rack in the roasting pan, spacing the pieces evenly. Bake until the breading is crisp and golden, 15 to 20 minutes.

11. Serve each fillet with a lemon wedge.

12. To save the catfish for later, allow it to cool completely; then refrigerate it in a sealed container. Do not freeze. Reheat the fillets by briefly crisping each side in a dry skillet over medium heat.

Chicken-Asparagus Penne

SERVES 4 (SERVING SIZE IS ABOUT 2 CUPS)

Calories per serving: 452

▸   SODIUM PER SERVING: 476 MG

Contrasting textures and layers of flavor combine in this pasta dish that's as gratifying as it is healthful. Mix things up by trying different pasta shapes, or switch out the oregano for basil. In place of the asparagus, try fresh green beans or broccoli.

8 OUNCES UNCOOKED WHOLE-WHEAT PENNE

8 OUNCES BONELESS, SKINLESS CHICKEN BREAST

1 TABLESPOON EXTRA-VIRGIN OLIVE OIL

½ CUP FINELY CHOPPED WHITE OR YELLOW ONION

2 TABLESPOONS MINCED GARLIC

4 CUPS SLICED ASPARAGUS

4 CUPS CHOPPED TOMATOES

1 TEASPOON DRIED OREGANO

¼ TEASPOON CRUSHED RED PEPPER FLAKES (OPTIONAL)

¾ TEASPOON SALT

¼ TEASPOON FRESHLY GROUND BLACK PEPPER

1. Cook the penne al dente, according to the directions on the package, with no salt added. Drain and cover to keep warm.

2. Rinse the chicken and pat it dry. Slice the breasts crosswise into very thin strips and cut the strips into ½-inch segments.

3. In a large nonstick skillet over medium-high heat, heat the oil until it's just short of smoking. Add the chicken and sauté, stirring constantly, until the chicken is lightly browned and cooked through, about 5 minutes.

4. Transfer the chicken to a plate and cover it with foil to keep it warm.

5. Turn the heat down to medium and add the onion and garlic to the pan. Sauté, stirring occasionally, until the onion is tender, about 3 minutes.

6. Add the asparagus and continue cooking and stirring until the asparagus is crisp-tender, about 8 minutes.

7. Mix in the tomatoes, oregano, pepper flakes (if using), salt, and black pepper. Simmer for 5 minutes.

8. Return the chicken to the pan. Cover and simmer until the chicken is warmed through, about 2 minutes.

9. Add the cooked pasta to the pan and toss to coat it with the sauce. Leave the pan on the heat for 1 minute before serving.

10. To save the dish for later, allow it to cool completely; then refrigerate it in a sealed container. Do not freeze.

Baked BBQ Chicken

SERVES 6 (SERVING SIZE IS 1 PIECE)

Calories per serving: 181

▸ SODIUM PER SERVING: 497 MG

Juicy, sweet, and tangy, barbecued chicken is always a hit at gatherings. Barbecue can spell DASH disaster, but the low-sodium, low-fat sauce in this version keeps things healthful. In grilling season, add some calorie-free flavor by brushing your grill grate with a little canola or olive oil and cooking the chicken over the fire.

3 TABLESPOONS CIDER VINEGAR

3 TABLESPOONS WORCESTERSHIRE SAUCE

3 TABLESPOONS NO-SALT-ADDED TOMATO PASTE

2 TABLESPOONS PACKED LIGHT BROWN SUGAR

1 TABLESPOON CHILI POWDER

1 TEASPOON DRY MUSTARD

⅔ TEASPOON SALT

½ TEASPOON FRESHLY GROUND BLACK PEPPER

½ CUP LOW-SODIUM CHICKEN BROTH

2 BONELESS, SKINLESS CHICKEN BREASTS, FAT TRIMMED

2 BONELESS, SKINLESS CHICKEN THIGHS, FAT TRIMMED

2 SKINLESS CHICKEN DRUMSTICKS, FAT TRIMMED

1. Preheat the oven to 350°F.

2. Place a wire rack in a roasting pan.

3. In a small saucepan over medium heat, whisk together the vinegar, Worcestershire sauce, tomato paste, brown sugar, chili powder, mustard, salt, pepper, and broth. Simmer, stirring occasionally, until the sauce thickens slightly, about 10 minutes.

4. Remove the pot from the heat and allow the sauce to cool for 10 minutes.

5. Rinse the chicken and pat it dry.

6. In a large bowl, pour the sauce over the chicken. Toss to coat the chicken thoroughly.

7. Transfer the chicken to the rack in the roasting pan, spacing the pieces evenly. If there is any sauce left over in the bowl, spoon it onto the chicken.

8. Bake the chicken for 30 minutes. Check for doneness by making a small puncture with a knife in the largest thigh. If the juice does not run clear, continue baking, and check the chicken every 5 minutes until it is done, up to 1 hour total.

9. Remove the pan from the oven and allow the chicken to rest for 5 minutes before serving.

10. To save the chicken for later, allow it to cool completely; then refrigerate or freeze it in a sealed container.

Crispy Thanksgiving Turkey Fillets

SERVES 4 (SERVING SIZE IS 1 FILLET)

Calories per serving: 220

▶ SODIUM PER SERVING: 510 MG

You can enjoy the flavors of Thanksgiving without the hassle of roasting a whole turkey. But the fact is that turkey breast is tasty and healthful any time of year. These crusted fillets may even tame your cravings when you're longing for fried chicken. For the cornbread in this recipe, use the Jalapeño Cornbread recipe in Chapter Nine, but make it without the jalapeños.

4 (3-OUNCE) BONELESS, SKINLESS TURKEY BREAST FILLETS
1 CUP 1 PERCENT BUTTERMILK
1 TEASPOON DRY MUSTARD
1 TABLESPOON MINCED WHITE OR YELLOW ONION
1 (4-BY-4-INCH) SQUARE CORNBREAD
1 TABLESPOON MINCED FRESH SAGE
1 TABLESPOON MINCED FRESH THYME
½ TEASPOON SALT
¼ TEASPOON FRESHLY GROUND BLACK PEPPER
1 EGG

1. Preheat the oven to 300°F.

2. Rinse the turkey and pat it dry.

3. In a small bowl, thoroughly whisk together the buttermilk, mustard, and onion.

4. Pour the marinade into a wide, shallow bowl or pan and add the turkey. Turn the fillets over several times to coat them, and gently massage the marinade into the turkey. Marinate for 15 minutes.

5. Using your hands or a food processor, break the cornbread up into crumbs; there should be about 1 cup.

6. Add the sage, thyme, salt, and pepper to the crumbs and combine well.

7. Spread the cornbread crumbs out on a baking sheet and dry them in the oven for 4 to 5 minutes. Do not allow them to brown.

8. Remove the baking sheet from the oven and allow the cornbread crumbs to cool, about 10 minutes, then transfer the cooled breadcrumbs to a separate shallow dish.

9. Turn the oven up to 350°F.

10. In another shallow dish, beat the egg.

11. Using your fingers, remove each fillet from the marinade and shake off the excess liquid.

12. Dip the fillet in the egg to coat both sides, then dredge it in the crumbs to coat both sides. Shake off any excess coating. Put the dredged fillets on a plate and pat them lightly so the breading sticks to the turkey.

13. Arrange the fillets on a baking sheet, spacing the pieces evenly. Bake the turkey until the breading is crisp and golden and the turkey is cooked through, 10 to 15 minutes. Serve immediately.

14. To save the turkey for later, allow it to cool completely; then refrigerate or freeze it in a sealed container. Reheat the fillets (thawing first, if necessary) by briefly crisping each side in a dry skillet over medium heat.

Turkey Meatloaf

SERVES 4 (SERVING SIZE IS 1 SLICE)

Calories per serving: 253

▸ SODIUM PER SERVING: 422 MG

Moist, savory turkey meatloaf is wonderful comfort food. All the more comforting is the money you save when you buy ground turkey instead of ground beef. Make sure to read the labels and use the leanest grade you can find—at least 90 percent lean. The leaner the ground turkey, the higher the proportion of white meat and the less dark meat and skin it will contain.

1 TEASPOON CANOLA OIL

1 POUND LEAN GROUND TURKEY

½ CUP ROLLED OATS

½ CUP CHOPPED WHITE OR YELLOW ONION

1 EGG

1 TABLESPOON WORCESTERSHIRE SAUCE

4 TEASPOONS CHOPPED FRESH PARSLEY

¾ TEASPOON FRESHLY GROUND BLACK PEPPER

½ TEASPOON SALT

5 TABLESPOONS LOW-SODIUM KETCHUP

1. Preheat the oven to 350°F.

2. Use the oil to grease the bottom of a 9-by-13-inch baking pan.

3. In a large bowl, combine the turkey, oats, onion, egg, Worcestershire, parsley, pepper, salt, and 3 tablespoons of the ketchup. Use your hands to thoroughly mix the ingredients.

4. Form the turkey mixture into a 9-by-5-inch oval loaf. Place the loaf in the middle of the baking pan. Brush the loaf with the remaining 2 tablespoons of ketchup.

5. Bake the meatloaf for about 45 minutes. The internal temperature of the meatloaf should reach 165°F.

6. Slice into quarters and serve.

7. To save the meatloaf for later, allow it to cool completely; then wrap it tightly in foil and refrigerate or freeze it.

Pork Scaloppini with Apple-Raisin Compote

SERVES 4 (SERVING SIZE IS 2 SCALOPPINI WITH ½ CUP COMPOTE)

Calories per serving: 310

▸   SODIUM PER SERVING: 200 MG

No doubt you've been served dry, flavorless, overdone pork tenderloin. The virtually fat-free meat can be overcooked in the blink of an eye. But turning it into scaloppini can solve that problem. In Italian, scaloppini are pieces of meat pounded very thin, so they cook superfast and don't have a chance to dry out.

¾ CUP WATER

2 APPLES, PEELED, CORED, AND CUT INTO
    ¼-INCH-THICK WEDGES

2 TABLESPOONS RAISINS

½ TEASPOON GROUND CINNAMON

1 (2-POUND) PACKAGE PORK TENDERLOIN

¼ CUP UNBLEACHED ALL-PURPOSE FLOUR

¼ TEASPOON SALT

⅛ TEASPOON FRESHLY GROUND BLACK PEPPER

2 TABLESPOONS EXTRA-VIRGIN OLIVE OIL

1. In a medium saucepan over high heat, bring the water to a boil. Add the apples, raisins, and cinnamon and turn the heat down to medium. Simmer, stirring occasionally, until the apples are soft but not mushy and the raisins have plumped, 5 to 7 minutes.

2. Turn off the heat and cover the pot to keep the compote warm.

3. Remove the pork from the packaging. From the thick center of the tenderloin, cut 4 slices about 1½ inches thick, to yield a total of 8 slices. Refrigerate or freeze the unused ends for another recipe.

4. One at a time, place the slices of pork between 2 pieces of plastic wrap and, using a meat hammer or a rolling pin, gently pound them to a thickness of 1/4 inch.

5. Combine the flour, salt, and pepper on a plate. Dredge the scaloppini on both sides, shaking off the excess. Place them on a clean plate.

6. Cover another plate with a double layer of paper towels.

7. In a large skillet over medium-high heat, heat the oil until it is just short of smoking. Working in batches, put the scaloppini in the pan in a single layer and brown them on both sides, about 1 minute per side. Transfer them to the paper-towel-covered plate and repeat until all the meat is cooked.

8. To serve, place 2 scaloppini on each of 4 dinner plates. Top each serving with 1/2 cup of the apple-raisin compote.

9. To save the dish for later, refrigerate the pork and the compote in separate sealed containers. Do not freeze.

Spaghetti with Meat Sauce

SERVES 6 (SERVING SIZE IS 1 CUP COOKED SPAGHETTI
WITH ABOUT ¼ CUP OF SAUCE)

Calories per serving: 512

▸ SODIUM PER SERVING: 440 MG

*Lean ground beef is as low in fat as ground turkey, and sometimes even leaner.
Make sure to read the labels and use the leanest grade of beef you can find—at
least 90 percent lean.*

2 TABLESPOONS EXTRA-VIRGIN OLIVE OIL
1 CUP FINELY CHOPPED WHITE OR YELLOW ONION
3 GARLIC CLOVES, MINCED
1 POUND EXTRA-LEAN GROUND BEEF
½ TEASPOON SALT
1 (28-OUNCE) CAN CRUSHED NO-SALT-ADDED TOMATOES
1 TABLESPOON BALSAMIC VINEGAR
2 TEASPOONS DRIED OREGANO
2 TEASPOONS DRIED BASIL
1 TEASPOON FRESHLY GROUND BLACK PEPPER
12 OUNCES UNCOOKED WHOLE-WHEAT SPAGHETTI

1. In a large skillet over medium-high heat, heat the oil. Add the onion and
garlic and cook, stirring, until the onion softens, about 5 minutes.

2. Add the beef and salt, and brown, breaking up the chunks, for 5 minutes.
Use a slotted spoon to transfer the beef mixture to a bowl, leaving behind
the fat.

3. In a large saucepan over medium-high heat, combine the drained beef
mixture, tomatoes, vinegar, oregano, basil, and pepper. Bring the sauce
to a boil.

4. Turn the heat down to medium-low, cover the pot, and simmer for
15 minutes, stirring occasionally.

5. Uncover the pot and simmer for 15 minutes more, stirring occasionally.

6. While the sauce is simmering, cook the spaghetti al dente, according to the directions on the package, with no salt added. Drain.

7. To serve, portion the spaghetti into 6 shallow bowls and spoon the sauce over the top, dividing equally.

8. To save the dish for later, keep the spaghetti and sauce separate and allow them to cool completely. Toss the spaghetti with a little olive oil and refrigerate it in a sealed container. Do not freeze. In a separate sealed container, refrigerate or freeze the sauce.

Orange-Flavored Beef with Stir-Fried Vegetables

Calories per serving: 233

▸ SODIUM PER SERVING: 390 MG

This tangy-sweet recipe calls for hoisin sauce, which is readily available in the Asian section of your supermarket. Fragrant, sweet, and salty, the Chinese sauce is a common component in Asian marinades and stir-fries and is also used as a dipping sauce. Stir-frying is a lightning-fast technique, so make sure to have all your ingredients prepped and nearby before you turn on the stove.

½ CUP FRESHLY SQUEEZED ORANGE JUICE

1 TABLESPOON CORNSTARCH

3 TABLESPOONS HOISIN SAUCE

1 TABLESPOON LOW-SODIUM SOY SAUCE

1 TABLESPOON DRY SHERRY (OPTIONAL)

1 TABLESPOON CANOLA OIL

1 TABLESPOON MINCED GARLIC

1 TABLESPOON MINCED FRESH GINGER

12 OUNCES FLANK STEAK, SLICED AGAINST THE GRAIN INTO THIN STRIPS

1 CUP BROCCOLI FLORETS

1 RED BELL PEPPER, SEEDED AND CUT INTO THIN STRIPS

2 CELERY STALKS, CUT CROSSWISE INTO CRESCENTS

½ CUP SLICED SHIITAKE MUSHROOMS

1. In a medium bowl, stir together the orange juice and cornstarch until smooth.

2. Whisk in the hoisin, soy sauce, and sherry (if using). Set aside.

3. Heat a large skillet or wok over medium-high heat. Add the oil and heat until it is hot but not smoking.

4. Add the garlic and ginger, and stir-fry, stirring quickly and constantly, for 30 seconds to 1 minute.

5. Add the beef and stir-fry until the meat loses its redness, about 2 minutes. Transfer the beef, garlic, and ginger to a bowl and set aside.

6. Add the broccoli to the skillet and stir-fry until it is bright green, about 2 minutes.

7. Add the bell pepper and celery and stir-fry for 1 minute.

8. Add the mushrooms and stir-fry for 2 minutes.

9. Form a well in the center of the vegetables and pour in the orange-hoisin mixture. When the liquid reaches a boil, turn down the heat to medium-low.

10. Return the beef to the pan and mix thoroughly with the vegetables and sauce. Cook about 1 minute.

11. Serve immediately.

12. To save the stir-fry for later, allow it to cool completely; then refrigerate it in a sealed container.

Beef Tenderloin Mole

SERVES 4 (SERVING SIZE IS 4 OUNCES OF MEAT
WITH ⅓ CUP OF SALSA)

Calories per serving: 230

▸   SODIUM PER SERVING: 226 MG

The flavorings in this roast are typical of Mexico's traditional moles, chile-based sauces that are as varied as the cooks who prepare them. In the United States, the best known is mole poblano, which combines the flavors of chile and cocoa. The real deal includes dozens of ingredients and takes days to prepare, but this dry-rub recipe is quick and easy.

FOR THE SALSA:

½ CUP DICED PINEAPPLE, CANNED IN JUICE

½ CUP SEEDED, DICED RED BELL PEPPER

¼ CUP MINCED RED ONION

1 JALAPEÑO PEPPER, SEEDED AND MINCED (OPTIONAL)

1 TABLESPOON CHOPPED FRESH CILANTRO

1 TABLESPOON FRESHLY SQUEEZED LIME JUICE

FOR THE BEEF:

1 TABLESPOON UNSWEETENED COCOA POWDER

2 TEASPOONS CHILI POWDER

1 TABLESPOON GROUND CINNAMON

1 TEASPOON GROUND CUMIN

1 TEASPOON GROUND CORIANDER

¼ TEASPOON SALT

1 POUND BEEF TENDERLOIN ROAST

1 TABLESPOON EXTRA-VIRGIN OLIVE OIL

To make the salsa:

In a medium bowl, toss together all the ingredients. Refrigerate for at least 30 minutes.

To make the beef:

1. Preheat the oven to 375°F.

2. In a small bowl, combine the cocoa powder, chili powder, cinnamon, cumin, coriander, and salt. Set aside.

3. Coat the tenderloin with the oil. Rub it all over with the cocoa–chili powder mixture.

4. Put the meat in a roasting pan and cook to the desired doneness (12 minutes for medium-rare).

5. Remove the roast from the oven and allow it to cool for 5 minutes before slicing.

6. On each of 4 plates, arrange one-quarter of the tenderloin with ¼ cup of the salsa, and serve.

7. To save the dish for later, refrigerate the salsa and the beef in separate sealed containers. Do not freeze.

Beef Stroganoff

Calories per serving: 624

▸   SODIUM PER SERVING: 538 MG

Rich and creamy, this dish tastes thoroughly decadent. But the substitution of nonfat yogurt for the whole-milk sour cream traditionally used in stroganoff cuts about 15 grams of saturated fat and 75 calories from each serving. Yet, the tangy lushness of this comfort food is all there.

12 OUNCES UNCOOKED WHOLE-WHEAT EGG NOODLES

3 TEASPOONS EXTRA-VIRGIN OLIVE OIL

1 TABLESPOON MINCED WHITE OR YELLOW ONION

1 POUND TOP ROUND BEEF, CUT INTO 1-INCH CUBES

8 OUNCES BUTTON OR CREMINI MUSHROOMS, SLICED

¼ TEASPOON SALT

¼ TEASPOON FRESHLY GROUND BLACK PEPPER

¼ TEASPOON GROUND NUTMEG

1 CUP NONFAT PLAIN GREEK YOGURT

1 TABLESPOON WORCESTERSHIRE SAUCE

¼ CUP CHOPPED FRESH PARSLEY

1. Cook the noodles according to the directions on the package, with no salt added. Drain and cover the noodles to keep them warm.

2. In a large skillet over medium-high heat, heat 2 teaspoons of oil. Add the onion and cook, stirring, until the onion is soft, about 2 minutes.

3. Add the beef and cook, turning the cubes occasionally, until the meat is evenly browned, about 5 minutes.

4. Transfer the beef and onions to a bowl and cover with foil to keep them warm.

5. Turn the heat down to medium. Add the remaining 1 teaspoon of oil to the pan and sauté the mushrooms until they are tender, about 5 minutes.

6. Turn the heat down to medium-low and return the beef and onions to the pan.

7. Stir in the salt, pepper, nutmeg, yogurt, Worcestershire, and parsley and mix well.

8. Heat the stroganoff for 5 minutes, stirring occasionally; do not let it boil.

9. Divide the noodles between 4 plates and top each with one-fourth of the stroganoff.

10. To save the dish for later, keep the stroganoff and the noodles separate. Allow them to cool completely; then refrigerate them in separate sealed containers. Do not freeze.

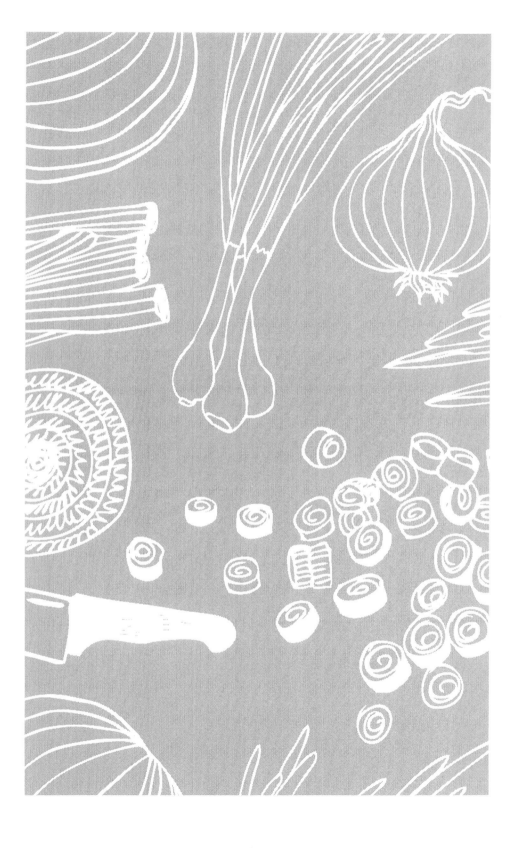

CHAPTER ELEVEN

DASH Desserts

Strawberry-Banana Frozen Yogurt

SERVES: 16 (SERVING SIZE IS 1 FROZEN CUP)

Calories per serving: 52

▸ SODIUM PER SERVING: 17 MG

Nonfat and low-fat plain yogurt are go-to ingredients in the DASH diet, especially Greek-style yogurt. Even in its nonfat form, it's thick and rich—plus, it has more protein and about 40 percent less sodium than regular yogurt.

3 CUPS NONFAT PLAIN GREEK YOGURT

3 RIPE BANANAS

2 CUPS FROZEN STRAWBERRIES, THAWED, WITH THEIR JUICE

1 CUP CRUSHED PINEAPPLE, CANNED IN JUICE

¼ CUP HONEY

1. Place paper liners in 16 cups of a muffin tin.

2. Put all the ingredients into a blender or food processor. Blend until smooth.

3. Spoon the yogurt mixture into the paper muffin cups and freeze until it is firm, about 4 hours.

4. To serve, peel off the paper and let the frozen yogurt stand for 10 minutes.

5. To save the frozen yogurt for later, take the cups out of the muffin tin and put them back in the freezer in a sealed container or a heavy plastic zip-top bag.

Frozen Chocolate–Peanut Butter Pudding Squares

SERVES 15 (SERVING SIZE IS 1 SQUARE)

Calories per serving: 113

▸ SODIUM PER SERVING: 174 MG

If you love peanut butter cups and ice cream sandwiches, this is the dessert for you. The recipe calls for white sugar and cornstarch, but the result is low in calories and sodium. So let yourself live a little!

26 GRAHAM CRACKER SQUARES (2½ INCHES EACH)
3½ CUPS SKIM MILK
1 TABLESPOON NONFAT MILK POWDER
1 TABLESPOON CORNSTARCH
1 TABLESPOON COCOA POWDER
¼ CUP SUGAR
¼ CUP UNSALTED NATURAL PEANUT BUTTER

1. Line a 9-by-13-inch baking pan with half the graham crackers.

2. In a medium saucepan over medium heat, stir together the skim milk, milk powder, cornstarch, cocoa powder, and sugar until smooth.

3. Bring the mixture to a boil, reduce the heat to medium-low, and simmer, stirring constantly. Cook until the mixture thickens, 3 to 5 minutes.

4. Blend in the peanut butter.

5. Pour the pudding into the baking pan and spread it evenly. Arrange the remaining graham crackers on top.

6. Allow the slab to cool for 30 minutes.

continued ▸

7. Put the pan in the freezer for 4 hours.

8. Remove the pan from the freezer and cut the slab into 15 squares.

9. To save the squares for later, remove them from the pan and freeze them in a sealed container.

The Original Flan

Calories per serving: 195

▸ SODIUM PER SERVING: 125 MG

This firm, eggy custard is very popular in Latin America, where it arrived with the Spanish conquistadors. Although it is usually made with caramel sauce, the original version—dating way back to ancient Rome—was made with honey. For the flan to cook evenly and gently, it must be baked in a water bath.

½ TEASPOON CANOLA OIL
1 EGG
4 EGG WHITES
1½ CUPS SKIM MILK
6 TABLESPOONS HONEY
1 TEASPOON PURE VANILLA EXTRACT
½ TEASPOON GROUND CINNAMON
2 TO 3 CUPS WATER

1. Preheat the oven to 325°F.

2. Move an oven rack to the center of the oven.

3. Use the oil to lightly grease the inside of 4 (8-ounce) custard cups or heat-proof bowls.

4. In a medium bowl, whisk together the eggs and egg whites. Whisk in the milk, 4 tablespoons of the honey, and vanilla extract. Do not beat the mixture enough to make it foamy. Set aside.

5. In a small bowl, thoroughly combine the remaining 2 tablespoons of honey and the cinnamon.

6. Spoon equal amounts of the honey-cinnamon mixture into the custard cups.

continued ▸

7. Pour equal amounts of the egg mixture into the cups.

8. Bring the water to a boil in the microwave or on the stove.

9. Place the custard cups in a deep 9-by-9-inch baking dish so that the cups do not touch one another or the sides of the dish. Put the baking dish in the oven and pour the hot water into the dish until it is halfway up the sides of the cups. Do not allow any water to go into the custard cups.

10. Bake the flan until the blade of a knife comes out clean when inserted in the center of one cup, about 45 minutes.

11. Serve the flan warm or at room temperature, or put it in the refrigerator, uncovered, to chill before serving. To serve, use a butter knife to loosen the edges and invert the cups onto plates.

12. To save the flan for later, allow it to cool completely. Tightly cover each cup with plastic wrap and refrigerate. Do not freeze.

Chocolate–Sweet Potato Pudding

SERVES 4 (SERVING SIZE IS ½ CUP)

Calories per serving: 172

▸ SODIUM PER SERVING: 92 MG

This delicious dessert combines the irresistible flavor of chocolate with the natural sweetness and nutritional punch of sweet potatoes. The potatoes make the pudding fluffier than gelatin-based versions. For a little extra decadence, serve it with a dollop of honey-laced nonfat Greek yogurt.

2 LARGE SWEET POTATOES, BAKED UNTIL VERY SOFT AND PEELED

½ CUP UNSWEETENED COCOA POWDER

½ CUP UNSWEETENED ALMOND MILK

¼ CUP PURE MAPLE SYRUP

1 TEASPOON PURE VANILLA EXTRACT

1 TEASPOON INSTANT ESPRESSO POWDER

½ TEASPOON GROUND CINNAMON

1. Using a food processor or a potato masher in a medium bowl, combine all the ingredients into a smooth mash.

2. Refrigerate the pudding for 2 hours before serving.

3. To save the pudding for later, refrigerate or freeze it in a sealed container.

Carrot-Raisin-Oatmeal Cookies

SERVES 24 (SERVING SIZE IS 2 COOKIES)

Calories per serving: 134

▸   SODIUM PER SERVING: 182 MG

If it's time for a treat and you can't decide between carrot cake and oatmeal-raisin cookies, these sweeties will solve your dilemma. To soften up the texture, this recipe calls for some white flour, which is on the foods-to-avoid list; however, per cookie, you'll get a negligible amount. For variety, leave out the raisins and/or add some chopped walnuts or pecans.

¼ CUP PLUS 2 TEASPOONS CANOLA OIL, DIVIDED

2 CUPS ROLLED OATS

1 CUP UNBLEACHED ALL-PURPOSE FLOUR

1 CUP WHOLE-WHEAT FLOUR

1 TEASPOON BAKING SODA

1 TEASPOON BAKING POWDER

1 TEASPOON SALT

1 TEASPOON GROUND CINNAMON

½ TEASPOON GROUND GINGER

1½ CUPS FINELY GRATED CARROTS

½ CUP PACKED LIGHT BROWN SUGAR

½ CUP UNSWEETENED APPLESAUCE

2 EGGS

1 TEASPOON PURE VANILLA EXTRACT

1 CUP RAISINS

1. Preheat the oven to 350°F.

2. Use 2 teaspoons of the oil to grease a baking sheet or line the baking sheet with parchment paper.

3. In a large bowl, combine the oats, flours, baking soda, baking powder, salt, cinnamon, and ginger. Set aside.

4. In a large bowl, mix together the remaining ¼ cup of oil, carrots, brown sugar, applesauce, eggs, and vanilla.

5. Fold the dry ingredients into the wet ingredients, 1 cup at a time until thoroughly mixed.

6. Stir in the raisins.

7. Drop the batter onto the baking sheet 1 tablespoon at a time, leaving 2 inches between each cookie.

8. Bake the cookies until they are golden brown, 12 to 15 minutes.

9. Let them cool on the baking sheets for 5 minutes; then transfer them to a wire rack to finish cooling.

10. To save the cookies for later, store them in an airtight container. Freeze if desired.

Fudgy Cookies

Calories per serving: 119

▸   SODIUM PER SERVING: 154 MG

You need chocolate. Now. Never fear, these fudgy cookies are here! Just two of them will satisfy the chocoholic in you. To soften up the texture, this recipe calls for some white flour, which is on the foods-to-avoid list; however, per cookie, you'll get a negligible amount.

2 TEASPOONS CANOLA OIL
¾ CUP UNBLEACHED ALL-PURPOSE FLOUR
¾ CUP WHOLE-WHEAT PASTRY FLOUR
3 TABLESPOONS UNSWEETENED COCOA POWDER
1 TEASPOON SALT
¾ TEASPOON BAKING SODA
4 OUNCES UNSWEETENED BAKING CHOCOLATE
6 EGG WHITES
1½ CUPS PACKED DARK BROWN SUGAR
1 TABLESPOON PURE VANILLA EXTRACT

1. Preheat the oven to 350°F.

2. Use the oil to grease a baking sheet, or line the pan with parchment paper.

3. In a large bowl, combine the flours, cocoa powder, salt, and baking soda. Set aside.

4. Chop the chocolate into small pieces and put it in a small microwaveable bowl. Microwave the chocolate at 50 percent power for 45 seconds. Stir the chocolate. If it is not completely melted, microwave at 50 percent for another 30 seconds and stir again. If necessary, repeat the process until only a few small lumps remain. Take the chocolate out of the microwave and stir until it is completely melted. Set aside.

5. In a large bowl, beat the egg whites until they are foamy, about 1 minute.

6. Beat in the brown sugar until smooth; then beat in the vanilla and melted chocolate until smooth.

7. Fold half of the dry ingredients into the wet ingredients until just combined. Fold in the second half until just combined.

8. Drop the batter onto the baking sheet 1 tablespoon at a time, leaving 2 inches between each cookie.

9. Bake the cookies until they crack on top, 10 to 12 minutes.

10. Let them cool on the baking sheets for 5 minutes, then transfer them to a wire rack to finish cooling.

11. To save the cookies for later, store them in an airtight container. Freeze if desired.

Heavenly Apple Crisp

Calories per serving: 240

▸   SODIUM PER SERVING: 124 MG

Gooey and crunchy at the same time, nothing beats apple crisp in the autumn, especially when you eat it warm on a chilly day. It makes a wonderful break-fast, too. When you bake this dessert, the heavenly aroma of cinnamon will fill your kitchen.

¾ CUP PACKED LIGHT BROWN SUGAR, DIVIDED

3 TABLESPOONS UNBLEACHED ALL-PURPOSE FLOUR

2 TEASPOONS GROUND CINNAMON

1 TEASPOON GROUND GINGER

7 MEDIUM APPLES, CORED AND SLICED ¼ INCH THICK

½ CUP DRIED CRANBERRIES

1 TEASPOON FRESHLY SQUEEZED LEMON JUICE

½ CUP ROLLED OATS

¼ CUP WHOLE-WHEAT FLOUR

1 TEASPOON GROUND CINNAMON

¼ TEASPOON SALT

1 TABLESPOON SOFT TUB MARGARINE

1. Preheat the oven to 375°F.

2. In a large bowl, combine ¼ cup of brown sugar and the all-purpose flour, cinnamon, and ginger.

3. Add the apples, cranberries, and lemon juice and toss to coat. Set aside.

4. In a small bowl, combine the remaining ½ cup of brown sugar, oats, whole-wheat flour, cinnamon, and salt. Stir in the margarine.

5. Transfer the apples to an 8-by-8-inch baking dish. Scatter the oat mixture over the top.

6. Bake the crisp until the apples are bubbling and the topping is golden brown, 40 to 50 minutes.

7. Remove the crisp from the oven and allow it to cool to the desired temperature.

8. Cut the crisp into 8 squares and serve it warm or at room temperature.

9. To save the crisp for later, allow it to cool completely. Tightly cover the dish with plastic wrap and refrigerate or freeze it.

Death by Chocolate Cupcakes

SERVES 12 (SERVING SIZE IS 1 CUPCAKE)

Calories per serving: 139

▶ SODIUM PER SERVING: 164 MG

Moist and chocolaty as can be, these cupcakes will make you the star of the bake sale. If they make it out of your house, that is. Be sure to use whole-wheat pastry flour, instead of regular whole-wheat flour, for a tantalizingly soft texture.

¾ CUP WHOLE-WHEAT PASTRY FLOUR

½ CUP PACKED LIGHT BROWN SUGAR

¼ CUP WHITE SUGAR

⅓ CUP UNSWEETENED COCOA POWDER

1 TABLESPOON BUTTERMILK POWDER

1 TEASPOON BAKING SODA

1 TEASPOON BAKING POWDER

¾ CUP STRONG BLACK COFFEE, AT ROOM TEMPERATURE

2 EGGS, LIGHTLY BEATEN

2 TABLESPOONS CANOLA OIL

1 TEASPOON PURE VANILLA EXTRACT

1 TEASPOON CONFECTIONERS' SUGAR

1. Preheat the oven to 350°F.

2. Place paper liners in the cups of a 12-muffin tin.

3. In a large bowl, combine the flour, sugars, cocoa powder, buttermilk powder, baking soda, and baking powder. Add the coffee, eggs, oil, and vanilla extract. Beat for 3 minutes.

4. Spoon the batter into the muffin cups.

5. Bake the cupcakes until a toothpick inserted in the center comes out clean, about 20 minutes.

6. Remove the cupcakes from the oven and let them cool completely in the pan.

7. To serve, dust the cupcakes with the confectioners' sugar.

8. To save the cupcakes for later, store them in an airtight container. Freeze if desired.

Righteous Pumpkin Pie

Calories per serving: 288

▸ SODIUM PER SERVING: 245 MG

What makes this pie so righteous is the combination of pumpkin and bananas. The result is sweet and creamy without the whopping calories or fat of traditional pumpkin pie. Pumpkin and bananas make a winning nutritional duo: Both are high in fiber, blood pressure-regulating potassium, and vitamin C.

FOR THE CRUST:

1 CUP ROLLED OATS

¼ CUP GRAHAM CRACKER CRUMBS

¼ CUP WHOLE-WHEAT FLOUR

2 TABLESPOONS PACKED LIGHT BROWN SUGAR

3 TABLESPOONS MELTED UNSALTED MARGARINE

COLD WATER

FOR THE FILLING:

1 (15-OUNCE) CAN PUMPKIN (NOT PUMPKIN PIE FILLING)

1 VERY RIPE BANANA, SLICED

⅔ CUP EVAPORATED NONFAT MILK

1 EGG, BEATEN

1 TABLESPOON PURE VANILLA EXTRACT

½ TEASPOON GROUND CINNAMON

¼ TEASPOON GROUND NUTMEG

½ TEASPOON SALT

To make the crust:

1. Preheat the oven to 425°F.

2. In a medium bowl, mix together the oats, graham cracker crumbs, flour, and brown sugar. Add the margarine and combine thoroughly.

3. Add water 1 tablespoon at a time, just until the mixture starts to hold together; do not let it become sticky.

4. Transfer the mixture to a 9-inch pie pan. Press it onto the bottom and sides in an even layer.

5. Bake the crust until it is golden brown, 8 to 10 minutes.

6. Remove it from the oven and allow it to cool.

To make the filling:

1. Turn the oven down to 350°F.

2. In a medium bowl, mash together the pumpkin and banana.

3. Blend in the milk, egg, and vanilla.

4. Add the cinnamon, nutmeg, and salt, and stir to combine.

To make the pie:

1. Pour the filling into the crust.

2. Bake until a knife inserted near the center comes out clean, about 45 minutes.

3. To serve, cut the pie into 8 slices.

4. To save the pie for later, tightly cover it with plastic wrap and refrigerate it or freeze it in a sealed container.

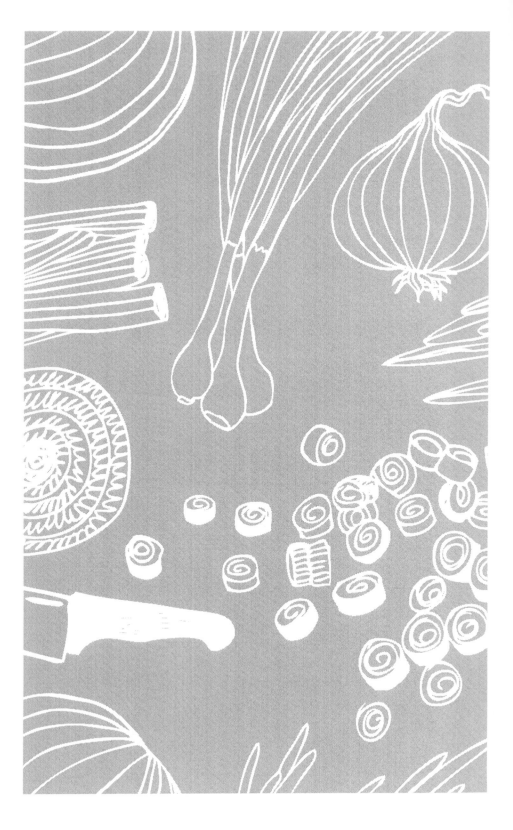

Ten Tips for Eating Out

1. **Do a little investigating and choose your restaurant ahead of time.** Stay away from all-you-can-eat buffets, prix fixe deals, and specials that might encourage you to overeat. Go online to look at the menu, and avoid temptation by deciding what you're going to order before you go. Call ahead to find out if the kitchen will accommodate special requests. Avoid restaurants that can't or won't prepare your food the way you ask.

2. **Don't be afraid to ask questions and make special requests.** Ask your server what's in the dishes that look good to you, and find out how they are prepared. Inquire about hidden ingredients that might not show up on the menu. See if there are any good DASH-friendly choices. Once you know what's in the food, request whatever modifications you'd like. Many dishes can meet DASH guidelines if they're made with less salt and fat. If there's nothing workable on the menu, ask if the kitchen will create a custom meal for you. Some restaurants charge extra for substitutions, but your health is worth a few extra dollars.

3. **If your order isn't prepared according to your requests, don't hesitate to send it back.**

4. **Find out if the kitchen is willing to make you a half portion.** If not, put half your food in a to-go box right when it arrives at the table—you'll get two meals for the price of one! Alternately, share your meal with one of your dining partners. The restaurant may add a split-plate charge to your bill, but you'll walk away DASH happy.

5. **Order two appetizers instead of a main dish.** You'll get more variety without eating or spending more, and you'll have a satisfying meal. Sometimes, the appetizers are even tastier than the entrées!

6. **To cut sodium from your meal, request that the kitchen leave out the salt.** Avoid foods that may contain hidden sodium, such as soups, casseroles, au gratins, and stuffed items. Ask your server to bring sauces, dressings, and gravies on the side. Stay away from olives and pickled or marinated vegetables; condiments such as salsa, ketchup, mustard, relish,

mayonnaise, and soy sauce; smoked or marinated fish, poultry, and meat; most deli meat; cured sausages, ham, and bacon; pâtés; and most cheeses. Fried, battered, breaded, and "crispy" items may contain a lot of sodium, too, as well as foods prepared with pre-blended seasonings or MSG.

7. **Almost anywhere that you eat, you can have a low-fat meal if you follow the DASH guidelines.** First, choose proteins and vegetables that are baked, broiled, grilled, poached, roasted, or steamed, and avoid deep-fried, pan-fried, battered, breaded, "crispy," crusted, and stuffed foods. When oils are essential to a preparation, such as in sautéing and stir-frying, request that the kitchen use monounsaturated oils such as olive and canola or polyunsaturated oils such as soybean and safflower, and ask them to use as little as possible. If butter is part of the recipe, see if the kitchen can use olive oil instead; likewise, ask for extra-virgin olive oil instead of butter for your bread. Select lean proteins or ask that visible fat be trimmed from meats and that skin be removed from poultry before cooking. Stay away from organ meats such as liver, sweetbreads, kidneys, and brain. Go for salad entrées with the dressing—or bottles of olive oil and vinegar—on the side. Or choose low-fat vegetarian options. Avoid casseroles and other dishes that might contain mystery ingredients. Have the kitchen leave off dressings, sauces, gravies, and grated cheese or put them on the side so you can use them sparingly.

8. **Incorporate whole grains into your meal when possible.** Request brown rice instead of white. When the bread basket arrives, pick the whole-grain offerings instead of white breads or rolls. Ask that the kitchen leave the croutons off your salad and the stuffing out of the bird. For pasta and noodle dishes, see if you may substitute whole-wheat varieties for white.

9. **Go for maximum nutrition by finding the fresh or raw vegetables and fruit on the menu.** Salad is always a good choice, with the dressing on the side. If you order pizza, top it with fresh vegetables instead of meat.

10. **And finally, there's dessert.** Try to limit the amount of refined sugar you take in by selecting naturally sweet fruit-based desserts, whether raw, cooked, or frozen. Pass on candies, icing, and chocolaty treats. Cut back on fat by ordering ices, sorbets, and gelatin-based items. Avoid whipped cream, ice creams, custards, puddings, and creamy or cheesy pastries.

Steer clear of baked desserts that contain a lot of white flour. And skip the cheese course. Ask if the kitchen is willing to serve up a fruit salad, even if there's none on the menu. Portion distortion can be a problem with dessert, as well; split your dessert with someone else at the table, leave half of it on your plate, or take half of it home with you.

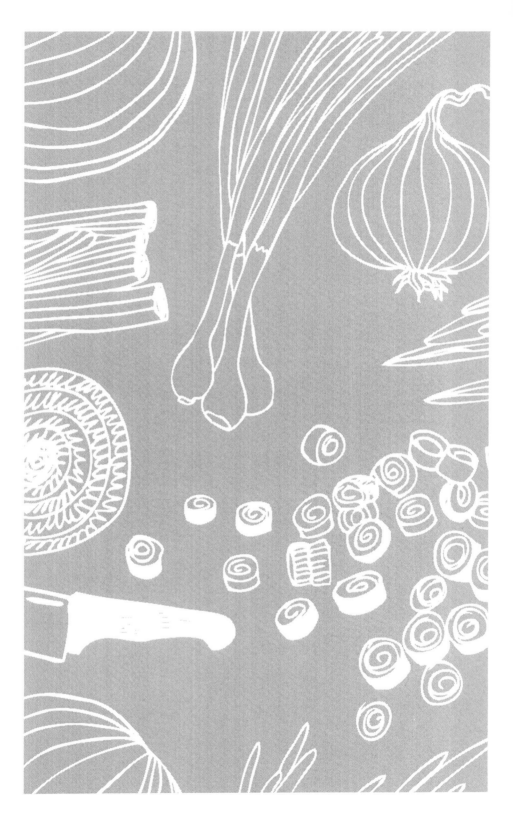

Thirty DASH-Approved Snacks

BREAKFAST ALL DAY

1 cup cooked oatmeal with 1 tablespoon dried cranberries
Sodium per serving: 297 mg

½ cup shredded wheat with ½ cup 1 percent milk
Sodium per serving: 60 mg

1 (1-ounce) piece granola bar
Sodium per serving: 75 mg

CRUNCHY DELIGHTS

1 unsalted brown rice cake with 2 ounces low-sodium cottage cheese and 1 ounce blanched spinach
Sodium per serving: 152 mg

2 ounces unsalted whole-wheat pretzels
Sodium per serving: 180 mg

3 cups unsalted air-popped popcorn sprinkled with chili powder
Sodium per serving: 2 mg

DELECTABLE VEGGIES

1 medium celery stalk with 1 tablespoon unsalted natural peanut butter
Sodium per serving: 150 mg

½ cup halved cherry or grape tomatoes with 1 tablespoon crumbled reduced-fat feta cheese
Sodium per serving: 207 mg

2 cups homemade lemon-garlic kale chips
Sodium per serving: 242 mg

FRUIT GALORE

1 medium maple-cinnamon baked apple
Sodium per serving: 4 mg

⅔ cup frozen banana slices with 1 tablespoon dark chocolate chips
Sodium per serving: 1 mg

¾ cup cantaloupe-grape salad with lemon and mint
Sodium per serving: 4 mg

HOMEMADE DIPS

¼ cup salsa with 1 ounce unsalted tortilla chips
Sodium per serving: 50 mg

¼ cup guacamole with ½ medium whole-wheat tortilla
Sodium per serving: 179 mg

¼ cup hummus with 12 baby carrots
Sodium per serving: 148 mg

¼ cup garlic-dill yogurt with ½ medium cucumber
Sodium per serving: 24 mg

NICE AND CREAMY

2 tablespoons homemade whipped cream cheese–sundried tomato spread on 1 (1-ounce) whole-wheat matzo
Sodium per serving: 149 mg

¼ cup light ricotta cheese with 1 tablespoon walnuts and 1 teaspoon honey
Sodium per serving: 56 mg

1 (12-ounce) vanilla-almond-oat protein shake
Sodium per serving: 65 mg

NUTTY STUFF

16 unsalted raw or dry-roasted cashews, pistachios, or walnuts
Sodium per serving: 0 mg

¼ cup unsalted raw or dry-roasted sunflower seeds or pumpkin seeds
Sodium per serving: 0 mg

2 tablespoons unsalted, dry-roasted peanuts with 2 tablespoons unsweetened dried cranberries
Sodium per serving: 4 mg

1 tablespoon unsalted natural almond butter on 1 slice whole-grain bread
Sodium per serving: 130 mg

SAVORY PROTEINS

1 piece (1 ounce) string cheese
Sodium per serving: 200 mg

1 large hard-boiled egg
Sodium per serving: 62 mg

2 pieces (1 ounce each) tuna, salmon, or yellowtail sashimi with a dash of soy sauce and ¼ teaspoon prepared wasabi
Sodium per serving: 115 mg

SWEET TREATS

1 ounce dark chocolate
Sodium per serving: 2 mg

1 (4-ounce) all-fruit frozen pop
Sodium per serving: 10 to 25 mg, depending on flavor

1 ounce (8 small squares) graham crackers
Sodium per serving: 175 mg

¼ cup chocolate sorbet with 1 tablespoon chopped salted peanuts
Sodium per serving: 65 mg

References

American Heart Association. "Salty Six: Common Foods Loaded with Excess Sodium." Accessed November 7, 2013. http://www.heart.org/HEARTORG/ GettingHealthy/NutritionCenter/HealthyDietGoals/Salty-Six_UCM_446090_ Article.jsp#.

Heller, Marla. *The DASH Diet Action Plan: Proven to Boost Weight Loss and Improve Health.* Deerfield, IL: Amidon Press, 2007.

Heller, Marla. *The DASH Diet Weight Loss Solution: 2 Weeks to Drop Pounds, Boost Metabolism, and Get Healthy.* New York: Grand Central Life and Style, 2012.

Mayo Clinic Staff. "DASH Diet: Healthy Eating to Lower Your Blood Pressure." Mayo Clinic. Accessed December 7, 2013. http://www.mayoclinic.com/ health/dash-diet/HI00047.

MedlinePlus home page. Accessed December 7, 2013. http://www.nlm.nih .gov/medlineplus.

Moore, Thomas J., Laura Svetkey, Pao-Hwo Lin, Nieri Karania, and Mark Jenkins. *The DASH Diet for Hypertension: Lower Your Blood Pressure in 14 Days—Without Medication.* New York: Gallery Books, 2001.

Moore, Thomas J., Megan C. Murphy, and Mark Jenkins. *The DASH Diet for Weight Loss: Lose Weight and Keep It Off—the Healthy Way—with America's Most Respected Diet.* New York: Gallery Books, 2012.

National Heart, Lung, and Blood Institute, National Institutes of Health, and U.S. Department of Health and Human Services. "What Is the DASH Eating Plan?" July 2, 2012. http://www.nhlbi.nih.gov/health/health-topics/ topics/dash.

Natural Standard Research Collaboration, ed. "DASH Diet." Healthline
Networks. Accessed December 7, 2013. http://www.healthline.com/
natstandardcontent/alt-diet-dash.

Nutritional Education Services / Oregon Dairy Council. DASH Diet Eating
Plan home page. Accessed December 7, 2013. http://www.dashdietoregon.org.

O'Neil, John. "A Diet That's Beneficial at Any Age." *New York Times.*
December 25, 2011. http://www.nytimes.com/2001/12/25/health/vital-signs-
prevention-a-diet-that-s-beneficial-at-any-age.html.

U.S. Department of Health and Human Services, National Institutes of Health,
and National Heart, Lung, and Blood Institute. *Your Guide to Lowering Your
Blood Pressure with DASH.* No. 06-4082. Bethesda, MD: NIH Publication, 2006.
http://www.nhlbi.nih.gov/health/public/heart/hbp/dash/new_dash.pdf.

Wellness.com. "DASH Diet." Accessed December 13, 2013.
http://www.wellness.com/reference/diet/dash-diet.

Index

R

Raisins
  Carrot-Raisin-Oatmeal
    Cookies, 196
  Pork Scaloppini with
    Apple-Raisin Compote,
    178–179
Raspberries
  Red, White, and Blue
    Parfait, 91
Red, White, and Blue Parfait, 91
Red bell peppers
  Orange-Flavored Beef
    with Stir-Fried
    Vegetables, 182–183
  Pepper Steak Salad, 102–103
  Southwestern Quinoa–
    Black Bean Salad,
    106–107
  Swanky Steak Sandwiches,
    128–129
Refined grains, 17
Restaurants, tips for eating
  out in, 207–209
Rice. *See also* Brown rice
  Pilaf Parmesan, 148–149
Righteous Pumpkin Pie,
  204–205
Romaine lettuce
  Chicken-Grape Salad
    Sandwiches, 123
Rosemary, 32

S

Sage, 32
Salad greens
  Swanky Steak Sandwiches,
    128–129
  Tuna-Apple Salad
    Sandwiches, 119–120
Salads
  Black Bean Confetti
    Salad, 143
  Bulgur and Chickpea
    Salad, 108–109
  Hearty Pasta Salad, 104–105
  Honey-Walnut Fruit
    Salad, 90
  Pepper Steak Salad, 102–103

Southwestern Quinoa–
  Black Bean Salad,
  106–107
Tuna-Apple Salad
  Sandwiches, 119–120
Tuscan Kale Salad
  Massaged with Roasted
  Garlic, 132–133
Salmon
  Fish Tacos, 121–122
  Teriyaki Salmon
    Stir-Fry, 166–167
Sandwiches
  Chicken-Grape Salad
    Sandwiches, 123
  Swanky Steak Sandwiches,
    128–129
  Tuna-Apple Salad
    Sandwiches, 119–120
Seafood, 14, 17–18, 41, 79
  Creamy Sole with
    Grapes, 164–165
  Fish Tacos, 121–122
  Oven-Fried Catfish,
    168–169
  Teriyaki Salmon
    Stir-Fry, 166–167
  Tuna-Apple Salad
    Sandwiches, 119–120
Seeds, 14–15, 18
Shopping list, 55–58, 67–70,
  79–83
Shopping tips, 26–27, 44–47
Side dishes, 47, 59, 71, 83, 132–155
  Aromatic Almond
    Couscous, 147
  Asian Noodles, 150–151
  Black Bean Confetti
    Salad, 143
  Brown Rice Pilaf, 144–145
  Cinnamon-Roasted
    Glazed Carrots, 139–140
  Jalapeño Cornbread, 154–155
  Lemony Roasted
    Broccoli, 138
  Lima Beans with
    Spinach, 137
  Maple-Pecan Mashed
    Sweet Potatoes, 152–153
  Parmesan-Crusted
    Cauliflower, 141–142

Perfect Coleslaw, 134
Pilaf Parmesan, 148–149
Spanish-Style Sauté Baby
  Spinach, 135–136
Tuscan Kale Salad
  Massaged with Roasted
  Garlic, 132–133
Zesty Quinoa, 146
Snacks, 16, 211–214
Snow peas
  Teriyaki Salmon
    Stir-Fry, 166–167
Sodium, 1, 20–21
Soups
  Creamy Butternut-Apple
    Soup, 110–111
  Turkey Noodle Soup, 112–113
  Southwestern Quinoa–Black
    Bean Salad, 106–107
Spaghetti with Meat
  Sauce, 180–181
Spanish-Style Sauté Baby
  Spinach, 135–136
Spinach
  Lima Beans with
    Spinach, 137
  Mediterranean Spinach
    Omelet, 96
  Spanish-Style Sautéed
    Baby Spinach, 135–136
Stew, Traditional Beef, 114–115
Stir-fries
  Orange-Flavored Beef
    with Stir-Fried
    Vegetables, 182–183
  Teriyaki Salmon
    Stir-Fry, 166–167
Strawberries
  Honey-Walnut Fruit
    Salad, 90
  Strawberry-Banana Frozen
    Yogurt, 190
  Tropical Strawberry
    Shake, 88
Sunflower seeds
  Granola, Pecan and, 93
Swanky Steak Sandwiches,
  128–129
Sweet potatoes, 152
  Chocolate–Sweet Potato
    Pudding, 195